Music to Help Overcome C... cer

The complete soundtrack of the pieces mentioned in this book and included on the album "Sounds for the Soul", *is available at:*
www.minjungkym.com

Cover :
Alain Toledano and Min-Jung Kym, Paris (France), 2021.
Photo © Anne-Sophie Soudoplatoff.

www.editions-hermann.fr

ISBN: 979 1 0370 3182 2

Min-Jung KYM & Dr Alain TOLEDANO

MUSIC TO HELP OVERCOME CANCER

The healing benefits of complementary medicine

Foreword by Adam Perlman

Translated from the French by Laurie Hurwitz

hermann

Depuis 1876

"Music produces a kind of pleasure which human nature cannot do without."

CONFUCIUS

FOREWORD

By Adam Perlman (MD, MPH)

> "Music can heal the wounds which medicine cannot touch."
>
> Debasish Mridha

Despite the amazing advances of modern medicine, cancer continues to effect over 19 million people worldwide and is the second leading cause of death. Receiving a diagnosis of cancer starts a person on a journey. That journey for most includes multiple doctors' visits and treatments, including surgery and powerful medications that can wreak havoc on the body while trying to find and destroy the cancer. The journey also includes a mix of powerful emotions from fear and sadness to hope and for some joy. The cancer journey can also be filled with a profound loss of a sense of control. This often and understandably leads people with cancer to look for ways to support themselves through their cancer journey not only to increase their chances to beat this terrible disease but to also support their quality of life while undergoing treatment and gain an increased sense of control, which in and of itself can be therapeutic.

This book is an important read for anyone seeking to support themself or their loved one through a cancer journey and in particular to use the power of music as a source of that support. The recognition of the power of music to heal both the body and the soul goes back to the earliest times of medicine and mythology. Since the time of Pythagoras, music and healing have been inextricably linked. Yet that link is typically not recognized in our conventional medical healthcare systems. Through the partnership and perspective of the two authors, Min-Jung Kym, a professional pianist who has had both breast cancer and colon cancer and Dr. Alain Toledano, a leading oncologist at the Institut Rafaël in Paris committed to providing his patients with not only cutting edge conventional care but also hope and relief of suffering through complementary care, the book provides practical guidance on how to integrate music and other complementary modalities in order to support both hope and healing.

However, this book is not just for patients and their loved ones but also an important read for health professionals who want to better understand and support their patients through their cancer journey. Through personal stories and as well as a review of the science, readers will gain a deep appreciation for not only the importance of music but other complementary modalities. They will come to better understand the role of what is now often referred to as Integrative Medicine in supporting patients with cancer.

During my 25 plus years as a board-certified Internist practicing Integrative Medicine and having had the honor of supporting many patients dealing with cancer at institutions like Duke University and now at Mayo Clinic in Jacksonville, Florida, I've personally experienced countless examples of the powerful role Integrative medicine can play in support of health and healing. When I began my career over 25 years ago, Integrative Medicine was a foreign term to most patients and healthcare providers. Now, worldwide do we not only have leading Institutions such as the Institut Rafaël in Paris but also organizations such as the Academic Consortium for Integrative Medicine and Health to which more than half of the Academic Institutions in North America belong. These Institutions include not only Mayo Clinic and Duke, but others such as Stanford, Harvard, Georgetown and Johns Hopkins to name just a few. Similar groups exist across Europe, East Asia and the world.

The growth in Integrative Medicine is being driven by a growth in the science supporting Integrative or complementary modalities. There is a growing body of science studying modalities such as music but also acupuncture, massage, mind-body medicine, health and wellness coaching, nutrition as medicine and more. The growth is also coming from a demand and desire by patients. Patients are seeking not only the best in conventional care but also a more whole person or patient-centred approach to care, that seeks to support the individual on a physical, mental, emotional and spiritual level. This is evidence-based medicine. Medicine that takes into consideration the relevant scientific evidence coupled with clinical judgement and a patients' preferences and values. It is medicine that seeks to not only treat disease or pathophysiology but to also address the totality of the experience of dealing with a diagnosis such as cancer.

At Mayo Clinic we practice medicine based on the motto, "the needs of the patient come first". We recognize that those needs extend beyond the treatment of disease. This book, by bringing together the perspectives of a patient who used music as well as other modalities as an adjunct to conventional care to support herself through two cancer diagnoses, with that of a caring and compassionate Oncologist, provides the reader, whether a patient, loved one or healthcare provider with unique yet practical insights on how best to support the needs of a patient dealing with cancer throughout their cancer journey.

Yours in good health,

ADAM PERLMAN,
2023-05-04.

***

Introduction

"You have cancer" – words we fear and don't ever wish to hear. Words that create anxiety, that forecast difficult months, even years, of treatments with serious side effects – a life entirely taken over by the disease. We sense the body is suffering and will be profoundly altered. We picture relatives who will be devastated, relationships that will be turned upside down, professional lives that will be disrupted, projects that will have to be postponed or simply abandoned. Not a single aspect of life is spared by this disease. And there's also the hypothesis of death that comes crashing down, into a life that until then, had been exempt from it. In short, your entire world collapses in the space of a few seconds.

Yet every year, it affects nearly 400,000 people in France and more than 19 million worldwide. Cancer is a common illness, but one that gives rise to feelings of profound loneliness. Its proximity to death still makes cancer a taboo, a disease that can sometimes make people feel ashamed, that they prefer to keep silent about. Too often, it prevents life from continuing to follow its course.

This observation encouraged us to write this book. The "us" refers to a professional pianist but also a patient, Min-Jung Kym, who has had both breast cancer and colon cancer, and her doctor,

Alain Toledano, an oncologist, radiotherapist and founder of the Institut Rafaël near Paris. This book was inspired by our encounter and our shared belief that in France, it still remains difficult for patients to find answers to their questions and to access to all the different types of care that can alleviate their pain and help them enjoy life again, despite the cancer.

In this co-written text, we wanted to set out a common understanding of the care pathway for cancer patients. With our combined experience as patient and doctor and also as a musician and music therapist, we explore ways that can make patients' lives easier, more than merely comfortable, by addressing the importance of the emotions we experience in the face of such an ordeal and the driving force of our relationships with care providers. We place ourselves firmly on the side of patients, their journey and needs. Intertwined with narrative of experiences from our own lives, this book is meant to enable cancer patients and their families to set about themselves into the reality of a cancer journey, to provide a means of continuing, despite the illness, and to give hope.

The main thread throughout this book is music. Music provides a basis to help deal with our emotions, for regaining hope and confidence. Through music, we can focus on the things that can make it possible to cope better with this disease.

Cancer is more than just a tumour, growths or diseased organs, and it's more than chemotherapy, surgery and radiation – all the things medicine tends to focus on. Without the treatments, of course, healing would be impossible. But the treatments alone are not enough.

Music came before language: the oldest-known musical instrument was a flute made from the bone of a cave bear around 40,000 years ago. People were making music long before our ancestors developed a complex language to communicate with. Does this mean, as some people believe, that music is at the very essence of our humanity? Is it music that made us civilised? It's hard to draw a conclusion; mammals such as whales communicate through sounds that are extremely musical. We know that while musical pleasure may not be universal, there's not a single population on the planet that hasn't created music. We also know that music stimulates the archaic areas of the brain, the ones involved in processing our emotions. Music's effect on the brain is becoming increasingly well documented, and this knowledge is used in music therapy. The emotional well-being of cancer patients has a substantial impact on their ability to heal, and music can play a crucial role in this process.

Throughout history, music and healing have been inextricably linked. In Greek mythology, Apollo was the god of music and healing. In ancient times, music had an essential place in health care and education. Pythagoras, then later Plato and Aristotle, believed that music had the power to cure problems of the soul or an imbalance in bodily humours. At that time, music was elevated to the rank of science, like mathematics, and was part of people's general education. Its ability to heal mental illness is evoked as early as the Old Testament. In the Middle Ages,

Avicenna, a Persian philosopher and scientist whose work had a strong influence on modern medicine, understood that the human pulse was musical in nature, and advocated the use of music for pain relief. The history of music and medicine are therefore very closely linked. Although it in no way replaces conventional medical treatment, music can play a very important role in healing.

These great thinkers recognised that the body and mind were not separate entities. With time, advances in science led to improved knowledge of the human body, leading to developments in medicines and treatments. As medical technology evolved, more and more lives were saved. At the same time, the technicalisation of medicine gradually led to a less global conception of both care and patients. Concentrating on the diseased organ and the nature of the disease left less room for patients to express their feelings, their suffering and their uniqueness.

But a patient is much more than a diseased organ. Patients are total, complex beings with their own emotions and values, their own physical and psychological needs. And they are asking for a health system that meets their needs; they want to be addressed as whole people, as a physical and psychological entity. This book is a defence of this approach: we want not only to concentrate on the illness, but also to focus on the patient's emotions. One without the other is insufficient. Desperation and unbearable suffering can lead for some patients to try alternative therapies – they secretly purchase vitamin therapies over the internet but don't dare tell their doctors. The need for hope is an anchor that shouldn't be overlooked. Cancer treatments are extremely long and difficult, and it's essential to give patients ways to manage their pain, to accompany them so they have a better quality of life despite the illness. Because this, too, is the doctor's objective – to treat the person, not just the disease.

This philosophy is what led Alain Toledano to establish his own Integrative care centre, the Institut Rafaël in France: to provide patients with whatever can help them live better, to hold onto hope in spite of their illness. Music provides hope and solace. A wide range of health care programmes are called "supportive care" or "comfort care" because they improve quality of life. We prefer to call it "complementary care", because it's used together and alongside medical care and encourages healing. We're certainly not suggesting that it's a miracle cure – there's no such thing. It is important to underline that this does not replace conventional medecine, but the most effective approach can be the one that takes patients and their needs into account. This does exist, and it's within reach for cancer patients and those around them. That's what we hope to demonstrate in this book.

The book also refers to tracks from a CD[1] with the selection of works that Min-Jung Kym played and listened to throughout her treatment, and that helped her to overcome her illness. She analysed each of them in terms of why and how it helped her. Surviving cancer involves accepting your emotions

1. Min-Jung Kym, *Sounds for the Soul* (Steinway & Sons, 2021).

and finding inner peace despite the physical and emotional turmoil, so we begin with a composition by Schubert that illustrates the healing power of music.

Schubert, *Impromptu Op. 90, No. 3*: finding calm
"This work by Schubert is very special to me. Schubert composed it the year before he died, when he was still very young and already ill. Like many of the pieces he wrote during this period, it has an extremely personal quality. These compositions announced the end of his life as an artist. I can't help asking myself if this composition was a kind of spiritual prayer for him. It is written in the rarely used key of G-flat major. A key that is soft but rich. Both these elements sing through in an almost endless lyrical flow of melody from start to finish, interspersed by rumblings of musical thunder, but what Schubert creates in the transition of harmonies is pure magic. This make us respond emotionally, transporting us into the meditative "Ave Maria" with which this work is often associated. I think of this impromptu as a musical prayer. It's one of the most lyrical works ever written for the piano.
This piece evoked strong emotions in me both when I listened to it and when I played it for myself, especially after I was diagnosed with cancer. At the time, it wasn't sadness; I was entering a period of reflection, of contemplation, thinking about what was happening to me, trying to make sense of my diagnosis. It helped me come to terms with the disease and find a way forward, which is why I included it on my album. I continue to play it today."

Min-Jung Kym

I.

Cancer in everyday life; living with the disease

1.

Using music to ease your suffering

Unexpected and long-lasting side effects

"Chemotherapy made my skin so thin that my sense of touch was impaired. I also had pain in my joints. These are just a few of the little-known side effects of chemotherapy: changes in sensation, tingling, pins and needles. In my case, they were particularly severe. I lost my connection to the piano keys.
In order to keep playing, I had to experiment with new techniques and adjust my way of playing. I saw it as a challenge and was motivated by the pedagogic aspect of learning how to adapt. Like a sportsman after an injury. Even today, although it's been three years since I stopped chemotherapy, this new way of working is still an inherent part of my practice."

Min-Jung Kym

Cancer affects more than the organs of those afflicted with it. Overcoming cancer can also mean undergoing surgery and aggressive treatments. It can mean living with the multiple side effects of these treatments for several months, often several years, because cancer is a chronic disease. There's more than just physical suffering – the patient's whole life is turned upside down.

Thanks to the work carried out by patient advocacy groups and research organisations, the side effects of cancer treatments are better understood. Managing them is an important part of cancer care, both to improve your quality of life and to increase your body's capacity to heal.

When you have cancer, there are many things you can do that can help to live as well as you can. It's not advisable to put your life on hold during the illness, and in any case, it's not even possible. The emotional power of music offers many ways to ease your suffering and provides an important escape from long-term illness.

Improving patients' quality of life, a vital necessity

In the past twenty years or so, the annual number of breast cancer cases has almost doubled, with 58,400 cases detected in 2018 compared to 29,970 in 1990[2]. At the same time, the mortality rate has continued to decline. Treatment for breast cancer is getting better and better, but according to Santé publique France, France's national public health agency, it remains the leading cause of cancer death in women. Several treatments can be used to cure breast cancer: surgery, chemotherapy, radiotherapy, hormone therapy – aimed at preventing female

2. See "National estimates of cancer incidence and mortality in metropolitan France between 1990 and 2018", a collective study by Francim (the French network of cancer registries), Hospices Civils de Lyon (HCL), Santé publique France (the French national public health agency) and Institut National du Cancer (INCa), July 2019.

hormones from stimulating cancer cell growth – and targeted therapies – drugs that target specific cancer cells without affecting normal cells.

Each treatment is tailored to the patient's specific type of cancer. Sometimes one treatment is enough, but often several treatments have to be combined and are spread out over several months. Between the screening and the end of the treatments, four months to a year may pass. These therapies all have in common the fact that they're very strong, with severe side effects that are difficult for patients to bear. This is a journey that requires endurance, a journey during which you may feel less feminine, less maternal, less attractive.

Some side effects are long-lasting and linger long after the cancer has gone. According to the French league against cancer, five years after the cancer diagnosis, 63.5% of patients still suffer from after-effects, and of those, more than half (56.5%) still feel tired and 73% say they experienced pain in the last two weeks[3]. Five years – that's the length of time after which cancer is considered to be cured. During the five years following their diagnosis, patients still have to undergo closely monitored treatment. Every year without cancer is considered a victory, and the cancer remains very present in patients' minds long after the treatment has ended.

3. "Five years after a cancer diagnosis, quality of life and employment status remain strongly impacted," VICAN-5 collective study, INCa, June 2018.

An altered sense of identity

Hair loss, nausea, breast removal – the most common effects of breast cancer are well-known, and they have been widely documented and publicised in the media. Everyone knows at least one woman who's been affected by breast cancer. But so much awareness of the disease can lead to trivialising it, to downplaying it. When reduced to mere numbers, cancer's side effects seem disembodied, abstract. People have heard of them, so they think they know about them, but the opposite is true. It's important to comprehend the enormous impact side effects have on a woman's relationships, her self-image, her sexuality. What are the consequences, and what do they mean concretely in the context of patients' lives?

Hair, breasts – breast cancer affects important body markers of femininity. Many women say they realised they had the disease for the first time when they understood they might lose their hair due to chemotherapy. Chemotherapy is a drug-based treatment that prevents the cells from growing and dividing. It works throughout the body, reaching cancer cells wherever they may be. It's usually administered intravenously but can also be given orally, in tablet form. Whether or not hair loss occurs should not be taken lightly in choosing treatments, in that some treatments enable you to avoid it. Hair loss usually occurs two to three weeks after the start of chemotherapy. But hair loss doesn't only affect your head and scalp; it can also impact eyelashes, eyebrows and pubic hair. It has also become a powerful symbol of cancer, perhaps the best known.

It epitomises cancer, and this can change the way others perceive you. Six to eight weeks after treatment has stopped, your hair starts to grow back. This takes time, and some patients are surprised to see their hair has changed, that it grows back differently. During treatments, they have to deal with this – whether or not to wear a wig or a scarf, or to apply special make-up.... This is an aesthetic issue, a dimension that might seem inconsequential. But patients need support with this; addressing such intimate questions makes it possible to cope better with the physical transformations.

Not all breast cancer requires surgery. Contrary to what most people think, we don't systematically perform a mastectomy[4]. In some cases, treatment alone can kill the cancer cells, and in others a lumpectomy[5] or partial mastectomy is enough. But often we have to remove the whole breast. Whether we perform a mastectomy or lumpectomy, the patient has to undergo a surgical procedure and anaesthesia, and cope with the accompanying pain and fatigue. In some situations, it's possible to perform a mastectomy and reconstructive surgery at the same time, thus avoiding the necessity for a second operation. Some techniques also make it possible to preserve breast skin and allow for a more natural appearance after the procedure.

Cancer may also affect a patient's hormonal balance; the menstrual cycle sometimes changes, becomes irregular or stops altogether. Breast cancer

---

4. Surgical removal of the breast.
5. Surgical removal of the tumour or "lump".

and its treatment can also have an impact on a woman's fertility, even leading to infertility. This can create a great deal of turmoil for women of child-bearing age. The French National Cancer Institute (INCa) estimates that women under the age of 35 account for only 10% of breast cancer cases annually, but this still represents nearly 6,000 women each year. In some patients, cancer and its treatment also cause early menopause.

Critical life choices

"One of my patients had just turned 30. She hadn't had children yet but wanted to have them. For her, the cancer diagnosis came as a terrible shock. In just a few minutes, she had to accept the idea of the disease and make extremely rapid life choices, choices as critical and basic as whether or not to have children. And all this while in a state of shock.

For us as doctors, such moments are crucial. We have to give our patients hope, reassure them, because there's a big risk they may refuse treatment. But we also have to explore every available option, because there *are* options. It's possible to preserve fertility. Few patients are aware of this, so few take advantage of it, but solutions do exist."

Alain Toledano

All these side effects profoundly affect your body image, your feelings about your femininity and your sexuality. You have to learn to live with a body you no longer recognise. A body that can be perceived as mutilated – which it is, in certain respects. A body that has changed as a result of treatment, because chemotherapy and hormone therapy can lead to weight loss or weight gain. These changes can lead to profound questioning. They can deeply affect a woman's self-image, the way she sees herself. Patients often express a feeling of injustice, even anger, when confronted with a body that is inadequate, a body that has betrayed them. A body that reveals itself as weak. Weakness for which there is often no rational explanation.

The body battered by cancer

Let's stop for a moment to consider the treatment's rhythm and the demands this has on the patient. After surgery comes chemotherapy. The number of sessions or cycles varies according to the type of cancer, but most often about ten cycles are necessary. Cycles are typically one to three weeks apart for about three months. Each session can leave you feeling exhausted for one to several days. This is followed by nausea and often vomiting, another well-known side effect of chemotherapy, one that generally fades at the end of treatment.

After a few weeks, fatigue sets in. Intense and pervasive, it increases as the treatment progresses. Fatigue often taken for granted by patients and their families as a normal consequence of any disease. But the extreme fatigue cancer patients experience is far greater than fatigue experienced in everyday life, and it can be very incapacitating. INSERM estimates that 80-90% of patients undergoing chemotherapy or radiotherapy experience severe fatigue. According to Dr Stéphanie Ranque-Garnier from the centre for pain relief at La Timone Hospital in Marseille, cancer-related fatigue has muscular and neurological components. There is no specific medical treatment for fatigue, but a growing body of research suggests that physical activity can significantly reduce its symptoms[6].

Memory problems

"People say that pregnant women can experience brain fog due to hormonal changes. Women can become a little forgetful, absent-minded... That's a little bit what happened to me during one of my cancer treatments. I was having more and more difficulty memorising my music. While I was used to having the notes at the end of my fingertips and knowing pieces by heart, it became more difficult for me to play without having the score right in front of me."

Min-Jung Kym

Without going into a detailed list of all the side effects associated with cancer, it's necessary to mention others that are less talked about but the consequences can be just as important. Joint pain, tingling, mouth dryness and mouth sores, lymphoedema (swelling), redness, digestive problems... The side effects are numerous, and as we have seen can cause lasting pain for up to several years. The list of these symptoms speaks for itself; when you have cancer, there are many possible sources of pain.

---

6. Léa Dall'Aglio and Vincent Guerrier, *Malades de sport, un remède contre le cancer* (Paris : Éditions du Faubourg, coll. "Pratique", 2020).

We have made significant advances in understanding cancer-related pain, but it's essential that we find even better ways to help patients manage it. Pain is an integral part of chronic diseases, and it is the doctor's role to treat the pain even when it isn't directly related to the treatment or the specific organ affected by cancer. Pain has both a physical component and a cognitive component. It's a symptom that in most cases can be treated with medication or appropriate therapies. Patients can easily express the physical dimension of their pain by clearly describing their symptoms.

Cognition is a vital component in the perception of pain and suffering, which has a psychological dimension. Pain thresholds (tolerance of pain) can vary according to the way in which a patient's emotional suffering is taken into account – suffering increases as hope dissipates. Not everything can be treated with drugs. By taking into account the patient's emotional state, we can propose solutions that make it possible to alleviate pain and suffering.

How life is affected

Without question, a patient's entire life is affected by the cancer and its treatment. These are all-consuming, and their effects on the body have profound repercussions on the lives of patients but also on the lives of those around them. Family and friends are invaluable in the daily fight against the disease – a fight that's best won when patients feel supported. But while the help and support of loved ones is crucial when people are facing this ordeal, the disease can also undermine their connection to their loved ones. Changes in the body and pain can interfere with a patient's sex life and relationships, and the loss of self-esteem can lead to withdrawal.

Family support is essential

"Chemotherapy began in September. One session every week, every Monday, for nine to twelve weeks. At the beginning, I tolerated the treatments reasonably well; I experienced few side effects. But three weeks in, the fatigue started to become more severe, more pervasive, and in addition to the physical fatigue, there was also the emotional fatigue that can be present when you have small children and it's difficult to make yourself available for them.

My family was amazing. For example, as soon as I started chemotherapy, my husband's mother came every weekend to help with the children. That support was essential."

Min-Jung Kym

Recurrent sick leave, the inability to work and in some instances disability, constant trips to the hospital for treatment, every week, every day, sometimes for months on end – the normal course of working life can also be disrupted. Leisure activities, relationships with others, everything life was made of before cancer can be disturbed.

Not only is your self-esteem damaged, but all this has a major impact on a patient's mental health. INSERM estimates that 40% of patients with chronic diseases suffer from depression. A feeling of anxiety arises very early in the treatment process. The disease is present from the moment of screening, even if it its name has not yet been spoken. This latency period, the waiting, is difficult to live with, and the uncertainty immediately incites negative feelings in the patient. Between the first questioning and the diagnosis, several weeks pass – several stressful weeks during which the idea of death has already emerged.

Everyone in the same boat

"I participated in a lot of group activities. Meeting other patients, being able to share information about our situations and our difficulties, helped me considerably. You realise you're not alone. For me it was a wonderful support system, a real source of hope."

Min-Jung Kym

Oncology now takes all these dimensions into account. We can't ask our patients with cancer to put their lives on hold, to disconnect their bodies from their minds. In addition, we know that by doing this, we multiply the chances of curing our patients. We now understand that it's essential to provide relief to chronically ill patients in order to help them maintain a life that's as normal as possible despite their disease. Even so, the process is far from perfect, and the patients' journey is far from easy. There's still a long way to go. But music is already providing us with answers on how to improve the quality of patients' lives thanks to its powerful effect on our emotions.

The power of music on the brain

Who hasn't had a strong emotional response while listening to music, feeling the emotions the music conveys in your body, getting goose bumps from it. Who hasn't felt that sense of community, of collective experience that can take hold during a concert? Music has the power to alter our emotional state. We often look for this in our daily lives.

Music is everywhere: in lifts, on the telephone to make the hold time less obvious, in stores to create a climate more conducive to shopping, in bars and restaurants to create a warm, cheery atmosphere.

As well as affecting our emotions, music is also a physical, sensory experience. Brian Greene, a physicist at Columbia University, defines a musical note as "a vibration that is very regular and repeats in a defined pattern"[7]. In fact, music produces "sound waves whose vibrations stimulate the whole body, in particular the skin's tactile receptors, but also the internal visceral receptors[8]," says Hervé Platel, a researcher in neuropsychology at the University of Caen. Music touches us deeply. It can bring inner peace, and it can help us express emotions that are hard to verbalize. We often talk about "frisson", about getting chills while listening to a piece of music.

---

7. Elena Mannes, *The Power of Music: Pioneering Discoveries in the New Science of Song* (New York: Bloomsbury, 2011).

8. Hervé Platel, "Pourquoi la musique nous fait-elle vibrer ?", in Emmanuel Bigand, *Les bienfaits de la musique sur le cerveau* (Paris: Belin, coll. "Cerveau & Psycho", 2018), pp. 15-26

Researchers from McGill University [9] in Canada analysed the neurological mechanisms underlying frisson. Their research showed it is linked to the activation of several pleasure mechanisms in the brain. We also know that music does not only act on the brain's auditory areas. Scientists believe that the auditory cortex, which perceives and analyses sounds, is linked to cognitive areas associated with memory and to pleasure systems in the brain. It's this combination that gives music its unique character.

Music and emotion

While we may not all be musicians, we are all music lovers. One might even say that we are born to love music. Babies around the world fall asleep to the sound of lullabies with largely similar structures and musicality regardless of the country in which people are humming them. What are the sources of this shared feeling?

Bach, *Arioso*: calm and reverie

"This piece is part of the second movement of Johann Sebastian Bach's fifth piano concerto in F minor. He composed it after writing his 1729 cantata *Ich steh mit einem Fuss im Grabe* (I stand with one foot in the grave). A feeling of purity and a quasi-religious dimension emerge from his body of work, and this concerto is no exception. It's normally performed with an orchestra, with a keyboard soloist playing the melody with the

9. V. Salimpoor and R. Zatorre, "Interactions Between the Nucleus Accumbens and Auditory Cortices Predict Music Reward Value", *Science*, n° 340, 2013, pp. 216-219.

right hand accompanied by a string ensemble. This reinforces its eloquent and solemn nature. This piece marks a small musical revolution; it's the first time the harpsichord was elevated to solo status. Until Bach, the harpsichord had always been considered as an instrument that accompanied; he turned it into a virtuosic solo instrument on the same level as the violin. Since then, it has maintained this status, as if in preparation for the piano's prized position in music.

This movement is perfect proof – if proof were necessary – that Bach, known as the father of classical music, had the ability to make the keyboard 'sing'. Bach was the undisputed master of counterpoint, the art of combining several melodic lines simultaneously. The part of the second movement that Bach called *Arioso* demonstrates this beautifully. The melody slips elegantly and tenderly into *pizzicato* (played by plucking the strings instead of using a bow). An arioso would traditionally be sung. Bach wanted the melody to be 'sung' the way a human voice would sing it. It's written in A flat major, a key that plunges the listener into reverie. This is a simple, serene piece whose slow tempo mirrors the rhythm of the human heartbeat at rest. It's extremely soothing and incredibly moving. I played it a great deal after my chemotherapy treatments. It brought me comfort and eased the pain I was experiencing."

Min-Jung Kym

"Music has charms to soothe the savage breast". This popular saying has a scientific explanation. We have seen that listening to music stimulates primitive areas of the brain, those involved in emotions. Researchers have shown that music has an effect on the production of cortisol, which is triggered by stress[10]. A high concentration of cortisol in the blood increases the risk of depression. Music therefore has a calming effect, because it reduces cortisol levels and anxiety or stress at the same time. But not just any piece of music can do away with your stress and anxiety. Those that have this effect are characterised by a slow, regular tempo and a harmonic, consonant melody. Could this be a coincidence? Researchers have shown that calming reactions are frequent when listening to pieces with a tempo of around 60 beats per minute (BPM). In classical music, this tempo is defined as "larghetto", moderately slow – a speed that also corresponds to the average rate of the human heartbeat at rest, on average between 60 and 100 BPM.

Long after Bach, Schubert composed lyrical pieces of purity equivalent to that of the *Arioso* analysed above with soft, flowing harmonies that also convey a certain tension. This is the case with his *Impromptu Op. 90 No. 3*, for example, examined in the introduction to this book. Its lyricism probes the depths of the human soul and soothes the heart. Its slow rhythm and its complex but gentle melodies bring pleasure and tranquillity.

Music's positive effects on the brain also have an impact on pain thresholds and on reducing stress and anxiety. Claire Oppert[11], a cellist and art therapist, described this in a book in which she recounts her

---

10. Stéphanie Khalfa, "La musique adoucit les mœurs", in E. Bigand, *Les bienfaits de la musique sur le cerveau,* (Paris: Belin, coll. "Cerveau & Psycho", 2018), pp. 83-90.

11. Claire Oppert, *Le pansement Schubert* (Paris: Denoël, February 2020).

art-therapy sessions with palliative care patients. She also explored this in research with Dr. Jean-Marie Gomas, who works in palliative care at the Sainte-Périne hospital in Paris. Their joint study[12], carried out on patients in intense pain during treatment, showed that "when the same analgesics were administered, pain and anxiety improved by 10% to 50% during treatments accompanied by music". Music's soothing effect extends to pain.

In addition to its relaxing effect, music also provides pleasure. It stimulates areas of the brain involved in the production of endorphins and dopamine, the "happy hormones". Listening to a piece of music activates what is known as the reward system, which allows the secretion of dopamine, often referred to as the "pleasure molecule". This part of the brain responds to biologically relevant stimuli such as food or sex but also to drugs, which lead in particular to the production of dopamine. Music is thus a pleasure in the most literal sense of the term, without risk of overdose!

Music and the brain

There's also a cognitive dimension to the effects of music on the emotions. Our capacity to appreciate or be moved by a piece of music is also linked to our education and our cultural references. Some studies show a kind of universality in the perception of

---

12. Claire Oppert and Jean-Marie Gomas, "Analyse de l'impact des séances d'art-thérapie musicale 'Pansement Schubert'", *Journal of Pain and Symptom Management*, Vol. 56, December 2018.

emotions conveyed by music. Don't babies around the world find similar nursery rhymes and songs restful and soothing, wherever they come from?

Nevertheless, listening to music from all over the world reveals significant differences. One of the most striking examples of these differences is the classic distinction made in the West between the major mode, which is associated with cheerfulness, and the minor mode, which is thought to elicit feelings of sadness. Middle Eastern music is mainly played in minor keys, which to people there does not express sadness; the emotional distinction we make in the West makes no sense there.

Music's connection to these emotions cannot be disconnected from the brain's cognitive systems. There is an experiential part to expressing emotions in which memories play an important role. Music is part of our lives starting at a very early age. Research even suggests that the foetus is sensitive to music in the womb. Our musical memories and the emotions associated with them are therefore shaped from birth, maybe even earlier.

Music stimulates many different types of memory – conscious, voluntary memory and also what is known as implicit memory, which allows us to retain information without deliberately trying to memorise it[13]. Working memory, used for learning, enables us to retain lyrics and to analyse musical structures, even if we're not musicians. Episodic memory allows

---

13. E. Bigand and M. Groussard, "La musique contre les troubles de la mémoire", in E. Bigand, *Les bienfaits de la musique sur le cerveau* (Paris: Belin, coll. "Cerveau & Psycho", 2018), pp. 141-158.

us to consciously remember music and the context in which we heard it. Associating an emotion with a specific recollection involves primitive, emotional, implicit memory. Music also involves procedural memory, which is both implicit and conscious, and enables us to learn habits and skills through imitation and observation; this type of memory makes it possible for us to hum. Finally, there's semantic memory, which allows us to remember and identify known melodies or melodies associated with events, consciously or unconsciously.

All these types of memory are involved with our emotions[14], and stimulating memory with music also stimulates emotions. It's this combined action of memory that also allows us to feel certain emotions in connection with music.

When listening to music, the strongest emotions, those that trigger frisson, come from changes in mode and tempo. Whether we are musicians or not, thanks to semantic memory and working memory, we are all capable of listening to a piece of music, of anticipating the way it may evolve. We may anticipate changes in mode or tempo, for instance, and this creates intense emotion. The context in which you listen to a musical piece, what you're going through at the time, the feelings you may have at that precise moment also play a significant role in the emotional response music evokes.

---

14. Pierre Lemarquis, *Sérénade pour un cerveau musicien*, Paris, Odile Jacob, November 2009.

***Reality*, by Vladimir Cosma: a "madeleine de Proust"**
"This song, from the soundtrack of the French film *La Boum*, ticks all the boxes for a hit song. The mechanisms of memory makes it timeless. Here's why.
One of the keys to writing a hit song is its structure: the verses, the refrain. The verse sets the song's tone and identity; it should be full of personality, be 'catchy'. *Reality* works well from this point of view – starting with the first notes, it captures the listener's attention. When this continues in the chords following, you're off to a good start.
The refrain, on the other hand, can be compared to the icing on a birthday cake: eye-catching, appealing, the part everyone remembers. It's stronger, more energetic. The verse leads us to it in a subtle progression. Then the music activates the part of the brain associated with memory – memory that learns the melody, memory that remembers the experience, memory linked to emotions. *La Boum* is a classic film from the 1980s that awakens many memories for those who saw it at the time. For this reason, *Reality* will always have a positive effect on people, especially to those born in the 1970s and 1980s!"

Min-Jung Kym

Vladimir Cosma, *Reality*'s composer, knew how to trigger emotional memory when he wrote it. With ritornello, the recurring passages, he awakened procedural memory in his listeners, who then felt happy listening to it. From thereon, each time to those for whom *Reality* has special meaning hears the song, they are filled with a sense of well-being, at least for the duration of the song. As we have seen, music can be a source of comfort and relief that can play a fundamental role in helping patients cope with cancer.

2.

Complementary care, at the heart of patient care

The accepted administrative term for it is "supportive care". It's not the prettiest term, but it covers an essential part of cancer. Supportive care is defined by law as "all the care and support necessary for sick people throughout the illness, together with specific haemato-oncology treatment where present[15]." In other words, all the care – in addition to treatments specifically related to the cancer – that can be provided to patients to improve their quality of life during and after cancer. This is no small matter, since as we have seen, cancer has such a profound effect on patients' lives. It isn't "comfort care" – quite the contrary. In fact, it's an integral part of the treatment for cancer patients, a complement to curative treatments and a leap forward, because it's now a patient's legal right, a right that was hard won thanks to the tenacity of patient associations and health professionals.

---

15. DHOS/SDO Circular No. 2005-101 of 22 February 2005 relating to the organisation of care in oncology.

Cancerology, the driving force behind the advancements in treating the disease

Everything really began in the autumn of 1998, when the Ligue contre le cancer organised the first General Assembly of cancer sufferers. For three months, 3,000 patients and carers spoke out at public meetings that this historic association had organised throughout France. After that, at the CNIT (Centre of New Industries and Technologies) at La Défense, 1,300 patients and carers met for a national meeting to review the current situation in the presence of Bernard Kouchner, then France's Secretary of State for Health. For the first time, patients openly expressed themselves about their experiences, their relationships with carers and providers, their requirements.

These general assembly meetings marked an important step in recognizing patients' needs and rights, even those beyond the cancer itself. They deserve credit for the 4 March 2002 law on patients' rights and the quality of the health system, which acknowledges the place of patients and the need to improve their quality of life. They also led to the creation of the French National Cancer Institute (INCa) and the implementation of cancer programmes in France that have made a major contribution to structuring cancer research, prevention, recommendations and care paths. Above all, these meetings helped to put patients at the heart of the system[16]. The first

16. Caroline Weill Giès, "La place du patient atteint de cancer dans le parcours de prise en charge : apport des plans cancer", *Revue française des affaires sociales*, 2017/1, pp. 176-186.

cancer programme highlighted the importance of a care pathway centred around the patient and authorised the existence of supportive care. Since 2003, three cancer programmes have been implemented in France. The last, completed in 2019, gave way to a ten-year strategy for cancer.

Thanks to the major advancements made in the early 2000s, we have gradually moved from a care pathway focused exclusively on curative treatments to a health pathway focused on patients, their needs and their well-being. The development of supportive care has gone hand in hand with the beginning of comprehensive patient care. This initially consisted of six mandatory components: pain management, psychological support, increased access to social services, palliative care, nutritional support and functional rehabilitation[17].

Today, complementary care encompasses a much broader reality and includes more kinds of care. The aim is to improve the quality of patients' lives, in every aspect during the illness. We try to focus on everything that can affect a patient's life. Patients' needs and their feelings about the disease differ significantly depending on who they are, on their personality, their history, their entourage. Complementary care is designed to be sensitive to this, and it's the carers' responsibility to keep a human, person-centred approach while

---

17. Philippe Colombat, "Les soins de support : état des lieux et perspectives", *Revue hospitalière de France*, n° 565, June-July 2015, pp. 32-36.

accompanying the patient, not to limit themselves to simply treating a disease.

Complementary care takes most aspects of a cancer patient's life into account. Starting with physical well-being: adapted physical activity, a specific treatment for managing pain and side effects with dedicated consultations.... These aspects of care have not always existed in equal measure. The beneficial effects these treatments can have are now better known, as is the positive impact of exercise, which is considered the only effective way to combat cancer-related fatigue. Numerous studies also show that this type of care reduces the risk of relapse.

It's been widely proven that complementary care improves the quality of patients' lives, but complementary care is also known to have a positive effect on their survival rate. Care that attempts to cope with the disease's after effects – such as preserving fertility, certain dental treatments or reconstructive surgery after a mastectomy – is likewise considered complementary care.

Patients may also need to be accompanied in their social, professional and administrative life. Sick leave, unemployment – it's not always easy for patients to understand their rights. In addition, the unemployment rate among cancer survivors has increased in recent years. More and more patients either cannot find jobs or lose their jobs within five years of having cancer[18]. Many cancer institutions

---

18. "Five years after a cancer diagnosis, quality of life and employment status remain strongly impacted," VICAN-5 collective study, INCa, June 2018.

offer social or professional support helping patients assert their rights and continue to work.

The need for psychological support is also more widely recognized today. Today, support for carers is also considered an integral part of this process. Because whether we like it or not, cancer is a collective affair. The support of loved ones is crucial in helping patients cope better with their illness. In addition, therapies have evolved considerably in recent years, with, for instance, art therapy and music therapy proving beneficial for patients for instance. New approaches are being integrated in complementary care with increasing frequency.

Responding to patients' needs

These developments have also been driven by patient demand. What we call complementary and alternative or non-conventional therapies are on the rise. Data differ from one study to another, but most estimate that 60-70% of cancer patients use complementary and alternative therapies. These are difficult to define and include a variety of healthcare practices that fall outside the scope of what is considered conventional medicine. Some are recognised, others less so. Some have what is considered a placebo effect, that is, one that is principally psychological, while others have proven their effectiveness. This can also be called as "soft" therapeutic medicine: yoga, homeopathy, hypnosis and osteopathy are among the approaches patients are increasingly turning to in order to cope with cancer-related ailments. Outside the cancer field, it's estimated that 75%[19] of French people have already made use of one of these therapies, in particular to treat anxiety disorders or manage pain.

It's difficult to categorize these practices because they cover such a wide variety of realities. Many of these therapies within approaches we call psycho-corporal, such as meditation and yoga; ancestral knowledge, such as acupuncture or Chinese medicine, can also be found in them. Some are more related to spirituality and faith, or to so-called "natural" treatments. These are regularly the subject of fierce controversy. In fact, evaluating them is complicated due to the lack of available data. And while some have been fully accepted and legalised, others are considered sectarian aberrations. In any case, they all have one thing in common: they respond not only to a demand from patients but also to an evolution in the definition of health itself.

Health was traditionally defined as the absence of disease or infirmity. Today, according to the World Health Organization (WHO), health is "a state of complete physical, mental and social well-being and not merely the absence of disease or infirmity". This new concept of health is matched by a broader vision of healthcare, one that is less disease-centred and more patient-centred. The inclusion of supportive care in the cancer patient pathway falls within this approach. Since medicine is the body of scientific knowledge and the means used to relieve, heal or prevent infirmities, injuries or illnesses, it is the duty

---

19. Claude Berghmans and Jean-Louis Torres, *Santé et spiritualité : un pont thérapeutique* (Paris: InterÉditions, 2012), p. 288.

of the healthcare provider to respond to a patient's needs – all of them – and to be concerned with the ways in which a patient may be vulnerable.

If we reject these practices as a whole, if we object to them too violently, we risk driving patients away from conventional medicine. Some patients may be tempted to abandon curative treatments, which, it must be remembered, are the only ones capable of treating cancer. It's better to embrace an approach that enables patients to adhere to their treatments and takes their suffering into account. For this reason, we need to integrate these therapies into a global approach, to set up a framework for them by including them in patient care. Because including integrative and alternative medicines also makes it possible to better understand these treatments, to encourage their use and to better inform patients. We can thus respond to a patient's needs by providing relief from suffering through therapies that have concrete beneficial effects.

From this perspective, the patients can then take ownership of the care project. Some complementary therapies, when combined with conventional treatments, have been shown to make a significant impact on the quality of a patient's life, and can become a veritable therapeutic tool that patients can rely on[20]. As we have seen, this is the case with music, which helps reduce anxiety and therefore lessen the

20. V. Suissa, M.-C. Castillo, A. Blanchet, "Le recours aux médecines complémentaires et alternatives (MCA) face aux incertitudes de la médecine allopathique", *Psycho-Oncologie*, Vol. 10/4, December 2016, pp. 272-280.

possibility of a patient sinking into depression. It's also the case with acupuncture, whose effects on pain have been proven, which is also the only therapeutic tool capable of preventing or treating hand-foot syndrome (redness and tingling in the hands and feet), a side effect of some types of chemotherapy. This kind of help can significantly transform the way people feel and experience cancer.

In fact, more and more health establishments are trending towards integrating complementary and alternative approaches in addition to conventional medicine, in particular in cancerology. Hypnosis, art therapy and acupuncture, to name a few, are already well-established in hospitals. This trend goes hand in hand with an ongoing evolution in medicine, which is now becoming more patient-centred.

Despite this, more than 20 years after this kind of care was first introduced, patients still encounter difficulties in accessing, and their demand is not being met sufficiently. There are major disparities depending on whether patients are being treated mainly by their private doctor at home or in a health-care institution or hospital, for instance. Institutions specialised in cancerology now offer a wide range of complementary care in their facilities, but due to poor information flow, the lack of coordination between private physicians and hospitals can still complicate access to these therapies.

Furthermore, the opportunities for alternative therapies are different in different geographic areas. The range of complementary care available in rural zones is often not as comprehensive as in urban areas, where it's easier for patients to find therapeutic options close to where they live. Information about the different types of care proposed in different locations should be shared among all the health professionals involved.

On a similar note, it's also difficult to understand the different types of complementary care that are available. Knowing where and in what context these therapies are offered can be daunting. Patient associations play an important role in this respect, publishing brochures and setting up websites filled with important facts, but the information is all too often not sufficiently communicated to patients or due to a lack of coordination between those in charge of the care project. For this reason, centres such as Mayo Clinic (US), and the Institut Rafaël centralises all the different types of care and health professionals under a single roof – everything and everyone together.

It can also be hard for some patients to pay for complementary care. In France, not all of it is reimbursed by the French social security system. Some hospitals and cancer wards offer complementary therapies for free, but not all; we more often see a decrease in public funding for supportive care. Today, mainly patient associations and some local governments are funding programmes such as adapted physical activity or psycho-corporal approaches. For patients who don't have access to these services for free, the out-of-pocket expenses can be high. This is undeniably one of the obstacles patients face in trying to get complementary care.

Finally, improved access to complementary care depends on listening to patients and enabling them to openly express their needs and problems. This requires time and availability on the part of health-care providers – two essential factors that are still cruelly lacking, especially in hospitals.

3.

Living well despite the illness

Music as a form of escape

"During treatment, I continued performing concerts. I continued playing the piano throughout my illness. Sometimes I needed to change my repertoire, I had to postpone my concerts abroad,but wherever possible, I never stopped practising and performing. It was extremely important for me to lead as normal a life as possible.

At each concert, I felt an unspeakable happiness, pure joy. It was like an escape hatch, a precious moment during which I could put the illness on hold. The audience didn't know anything about what I was going through. All I had to do was concentrate on the music. Those moments belonged to me alone. I was entering another realm where the illness had no place. I changed my musical programme according to the emotions I was feeling during the different periods I was going through: turbulent pieces to express frustration but also soothing pieces, the ones that made me feel better and that I also played for myself at home.

There was really an added dimension to performing live during that period, because music transports and takes you far from your everyday life – and because I was able continue practising my art, despite the disease."

Min-Jung Kym

The Bible tells us that King Saul, abandoned by the spirit of God and deeply agitated, felt calm only when David played the lyre for him. Since ancient times – long before we invented music therapy as it is known today – music has been used as a therapeutic tool. It has the power to fully immerse us in a different universe, to anchor us in the present. Thanks to its ability to engage our attention, it can create a secure framework outside the framework of the illness, at least for a few moments. Life doesn't stop during cancer, but cancer can take over your life. Music brings life. Music therapy uses this emotional power to develop a sense of trust and help patients feel safe, enabling them to let go of their illness. It introduces new, vital energy into a place where the disease has been taking up all the room.

For years, we have been refuting the cliché that cancer patients need to stay in bed, rest and severely limit their activities. A paradigm shift has occurred in that we now know that staying active and maintaining as normal a life as possible helps considerably in coping with cancer. It allows you to forget your condition, improve your quality of life and better accept the disease. Too much time resting and staying inactive being imprisoned by the disease can be as detrimental both to patients' physical health and their psychological health. But despite everything, this myth is still alive and well. All too often, we recommend that patients rest above all else. But as we've seen, cancer tends to be a chronic disease, and you must be able to live with it. Not just survive, but lead a full life, with everything life is made of, even if you have to adjust to a new way of life: love, friendship, family, art, music, exercise, work, all your daily activities as well as the little moments that belong to you.... This doesn't mean being in denial of the disease, but allowing the disease it to take its rightful place – which is already very prominent in patients' lives.

All the avenues we have explored in the previous chapters can enable cancer patients to improve their sense of well-being. This is what it's all about: living with the disease, continuing to live life despite the cancer. Complementary care gives you a number of tools that can limit physical and psychological side effects. They can significantly contribute to restoring quality of life, to lessening pain and suffering, relieving certain symptoms or helping patients sustain a sense of normalcy. But you also have to enjoy your life. This is a simple rule, but one that's extremely difficult to put into practice when you're coping with an illness such as cancer, with all the doubts, fears and pain that go along with it.

Celebrating the present

Cancer patients invariably confront an onslaught of fears. You might be afraid of dying, afraid of suffering or pain, afraid of your body will be altered, afraid your relationships with those around you will change... All these fears are very real and can prevent you from living life to the fullest. The idea is not to make patients feel guilty for being afraid. Fear is useful, natural and legitimate. It protects us and helps us survive. Identifying it, giving it a name and talking about it is already one way to respond.

But too much fear can result in anxiety, which makes it more diffuse, more difficult to identify, more difficult to control.

To reduce your fears, you need to fight against the perceptions associated with the disease. The first perception is connected to the anxiety of losing control of your body or your will to live. Patients are afraid of losing their dignity and autonomy. The carer's role is to help patients maintain their dignity and autonomy. The second is, of course, death, and what cancer represents in the collective imagination: a body that has become old, emaciated and weak. It's important to demystify this image and remember that sometimes, cancer is temporary.

Bringing life

"I remember one patient I was seeing for the first time. She had recently been diagnosed with cancer and it was our first appointment.

As I was explaining the course of her treatment, her mind suddenly seemed to be elsewhere and her eyes drifted off in the distance. I had been talking about chemotherapy and the fact that she might lose her hair. In a matter of moments, she froze. I felt as if she was no longer there in my office with me.

She may have known she had cancer, but the minute I talked to her about her hair, she stopped, as if monopolised by the disease. These are crucial moments in a consultation. If you don't pay attention to them, you risk losing the patient. All the patient thinks about is the disease, its side effects, the risks, and you are no longer in a positive interaction.

So I stopped talking. I slowed down, taking the time to look at her, to ask her what she was feeling at that very moment. We were able to talk about her fears, and I took all the time that was needed to listen to her and to try to respond. The consultation finally reverted to normal, and my patient was once again fully engaged in her healing process. It's our role as doctors to identify these moments, the times when a patient is fearful. We can then give them answers, remind them that the disease and its effects are only temporary, that solutions do exist and that life goes on in spite of everything. This is one of the things that helps give patients the willpower to live with cancer. When I succeed in this, I know my job is already partly done because I've helped engage my patient's survival instinct."

Alain Toledano

Changes in the body linked to cancer are mostly temporary. Even if the disease lasts for several months or years, even if the fear of recurrence remains in the patient's body and heart for years, the actual pain and injury to the body last only for a short time. Being aware of this makes it easier to accept what is happening in the here and now. The wear and tear of such an ordeal tends to push patients to project into the future. But then they are no longer in the present time; the disease takes all the space and undermines the life instinct. Patients may abandon their bodies to the disease, creating disconnection between body and mind. This can lead patients to be overtaken by the changes caused by cancer.

To prepare for a difficult event, which in the case of cancer can be death, people are often tempted to project themselves into a hypothetical future. All too often, we cling to the past; we desperately hope to return to our previous life, the one we consider normal, the one in which the disease never existed. We can be trapped in nostalgia, stuck in the past, or focus entirely on the future. But it's in the present moment that you find the vital energy that gives you the strength to cope with cancer. We have to face the difficulty of accepting reality. This doesn't mean that patients don't have the right to protest, to rebel against what's happening to them – on the contrary. Cancer is an ordeal, and there's no point in denying it. Accepting this is what legitimises all the efforts cancer patients make on a daily basis.

Céline Lefève, a philosopher, director of the AP-HP (Assistance Publique Hôpitaux de Paris) and chair in the philosophy of medical care at the École normale supérieure, defines living with a chronic disease as a "balancing act[21]" in that patients constantly juggle their vulnerabilities as they try to adapt to their condition. They use all their energy all the time to try to re-appropriate their lives and live normally.

But there's nothing normal about suffering every day. There's nothing normal about facing the risk of death every day. There's nothing normal about seeing your body battered by the treatments that are supposed to cure you, even though you know they're necessary. The cancer ordeal itself is abnormal. And all you want is to go back to the life you had before, the one you consider normal, rightly or wrongly. Curiously, it's when we understand that there will

---

21. Céline Lefève, "La maladie chronique révèle les liens affectifs qui nous tiennent en vie", *Le Monde*, 19 August 2018.

be no return to the life we had before, that cancer changes us forever. We can then concentrate on the moment, on the journey with the disease each day and on the life that is possible in spite of it all.

The difficult exercise of letting go

Carers have a role to play in this search for acceptance and for letting go. Integrative medicine has fully embraced this principle. By making a diverse group of carers available to patients, all the components of care in the broadest sense (of course medical, but also psychological or social) can be mobilised to keep them from feeling disempowered. An integrative approach distances itself from conventional medicine in that it tries to meet all the support needs of people with cancer, through all the practices that can help patients. It treats the whole patient and addresses all the different aspect of a patient's life in all its multiple dimensions.

Care goes far beyond the medical register. This is what's known as the ethics of care, and our goal is to draw on all possible resources that can help patients feel better. Some of these are widely known and accepted, such as psychological care, physical activity, body-related care such as physiotherapy or traditional medicines like acupuncture... But we also need to consider the fact that a patient's relationships with friends and family, leisure activities, work or creative outlets all represent kinds of care. All the means that can empower patients and help them take back their bodies and lives should be activated.

Music therapy, a tool for letting go

Mozart, *Sonata K. 331, known as "Alla Turca"*, last movement: lightness

"This sonata is recognisable from the very first notes. The melody is very simple, almost naive. This does not mean that it's without complexity; Mozart wrote it to show off his prowess as a pianist.

It begins in A major, a key also found in his *Piano Concerto No. 23*. In the beginning, it's intimate; you can feel the hesitation, and it ends in exhuberance.

The first movement consists of a main theme and six variations on that theme, each with its own character. Here, Mozart plays with rhythms, beats, hand crossings and key changes, including a variation in a minor key, expressing the fanciful quality typical of Mozart's compositions and his unique ability to tell us stories through music.

He composed this sonata during his oriental period (as with his opera *Die Entführung aus dem Serail*). In the third movement he wanted to evoke all the instruments that play in a Turkish miltary orchestra. This movement is suggestive of letting go. You listen to it with no arrière-pensée; it has such a festive tone, and enables you to leave everything behind. It makes you feel liberated. When you listen to it, you're fully and totally in the present. I started playing it and listening to it when I was halfway through my treatments, because for me it also embodied the kind of optimism I was clinging to as the end was approaching."

Min-Jung Kym

Music is a wonderful tool for healing your emotions and for letting go of anger and fear when you're faced with a challenge. Music therapy is therefore increasingly used to help patients cope with stress and promote healing. Although the vocabulary used in music therapy is rather recent, music and health have been associated for a very long time. In the ancient past, people used music to heal themselves. In addition to the legend of Saul and David, we know that the Egyptians utilised music to cure snake bites[22] and that Plato, based on Pythagoras' work on numbers, believed the ills of the soul could be cured through musical compositions[23]. From the Renaissance onwards, music was prescribed for treating melancholy and what is now called mental health in general.

Music therapy as we know and practice it today developed after World War II, using music to treat veterans suffering from trauma. Music was proved effective for people with traumatic brain injuries, neurological conditions or neurological diseases. "Combat fatigue" and post-traumatic stress disorder in former soldiers proved to be a fertile ground for exploration, and music therapy as a profession really took off.

Music not only soothes the ills of the spirit, but also helps to make the here and now more bearable through its ability to help people focus and keep them in the present moment. This ability, combined with music's powerful effects on our emotions,

---

22. E. Bigand and B. Tillmann, "La musique qui 'panse' les neurones", in. E. Bigand (ed.), *Les bienfaits de la musique sur le cerveau,* (Paris: Belin, coll. "Cerveau & Psycho", 2018).

23. François-Xavier Vrait, *La musicothérapie* (Paris: PUF, coll. "Que sais-je?", 2018).

provides us with valuable insight into helping people with chronic illnesses to live better in the midst of a particularly difficult situation. The goal of music therapy is to relieve the patient's suffering. Through music, we can try to establish a form of communication with the patient that enables us to elicit an emotional response.

In music therapy, we look for the patient's full and complete attention. Music makes this possible, which is one of the reasons why it is such a powerful tool for letting go. We play on music's rhythm in order to capture the patient's attention and create an atmosphere conducive to concentration. Most of the time, it's best to start with a rather slow piece that has a constant rhythm, something with a moderate pace, called "andante", like a walk, something almost hypnotic. Our goal is also to create a safe environment for the patient. Once the foundations have been laid, the work on their emotional situation can begin.

Depending on the response we're trying to provoke, we constantly change the music in an ongoing dialogue with the patient. The music's rhythm is of prime importance, particularly for young children but also for adults. A fast rhythm causes a form of excitement, while on the other hand a slow rhythm generates trust and reassurance. By playing on both minor and major keys, we can arouse different emotions. If possible, it's best to avoid pieces that are too calm, too relaxed, except at the beginning or end of a session. If the atmosphere is too soft or ill-defined, you don't connect with the patient.

There are basically two approaches in music therapy: active, in which the patients participate by playing an instrument or singing—whether they're musicians or not—or passive, in which the patients listen to music that will have an effect on them. Listening to live or recorded music gives patients a few moments of respite and distance from the disease and their pain. At the same time, thanks to the way music affects the patient's level of cortisol (the "stress hormone"), as we mentioned in the first chapter, music reduces anxiety, helping patients cope with feelings of loneliness, fear and stress. In active music therapy sessions, the goal is to enable patients to express their emotions; music is used as a means of communication.

In group sessions, although patients aren't necessarily asked to play instruments, they're encouraged to express the feelings or memories that may arise while listening to a piece of music, anything that can allow them to articulate their sensations, emotions or needs. Patients are also encouraged to talk to each other about their feelings, to share their experiences and impressions.

In all these situations, we look for a form of dialogue with the patient. Our challenge is to awaken their inner emotions without using words. We can use memory to encourage them to express certain feelings. To do this, we rely a great deal on tempo and frequencies (low or high). Playing the same piece in different ways, making it fast or slow, high or low, changes our perception of the emotions it can convey. High notes generally evoke something light and cheerful, while low notes bring up something deeper and calmer. Turbulent music can allow patients to let go of negative feelings by expressing them freely within the safe therapeutic context the music creates.

This makes it possible for patients to let go, to release anxiety and stress. An active, participatory approach reinforces this: by giving patients the pleasure of "doing", but also the confidence that comes from creating, which has an immediate calming effect. Music therapy can be seen as a tool for helping cancer patients, as well as people in other difficult situations, to mentally prepare their next steps.

The doctor's role

Doctors play a central role in this process and in helping patients maintain their future goals in spite of the disease. They must establish trust with their patients. Integrative medicine places great emphasis on the doctor-patient relationship; this is an essential concept in talking about care, one that is all too often neglected, which we will discuss in detail in the following chapters. Given how quickly time passes and the significant financial resources needed for medical procedures, we don't value enough the time spent and the investment made in the quality of the doctor-patient relationship, even though this is what both doctors and patients aspire to.

Doctors are in an excellent position to pay attention to their patients' fears and to provide answers that will help overcome them. As we said earlier, fear is natural – it protects us, and it's what makes us human. It's an inherent part of the cancer journey. But doctors must help patients overcome this fear, to keep them from suffering because of it. Very often, the images patients have of the disease and the ideas they carry around is what really frightens patients.

The doctor's role is to take the time to answer these questions, to make it possible for the patient to identify them, give them a name, talk about them. Patients can thus understand them, which is essential to finally ridding themselves of them. Establishing goals, allowing yourself to live life then becomes possible. Reviving hope alleviates suffering. In an illness such as cancer, we have no choice but to rely on others, and the care relationship takes on a vital role. It's one of the most important links in the healing process but also in living with the disease. Patients are confronted with a multitude of medical procedures and have carers. The quality of the relationship is essential if they're to be able to surrender—without losing themselves—to their therapies with confidence, in the hands of carers who look after them. And carers must spend the time needed to create and maintain this bond of trust. Acknowledging, listening to and responding to patients' fears and suffering gives them hope, makes them feel that life becomes possible again. This helps patients take control of their bodies, their lives and therefore their treatment.

Day-to-day

Inner resources

Cooking for better health

"I've always loved cooking, and have been passionate about it for years. it. Mixing flavours, taking the time to compose a meal, thinking about the wines that might accompany it... I love spending time selecting ingredients, learning new recipes, new techniques, chopping vegetables, watching over a broth... For me, cooking is like musical improvisation: once you have a basic repertoire, you can add new ingredients and improvise to create your own interpretation. In addition, cooking is not a solitary pleasure, and what I like most of all is cooking for my family, preparing big meals and spoiling the people I love.

When I had cancer, this passion took on a particularly important role. I remember so clearly how I reacted when I was diagnosed with my second cancer, even though I hadn't yet finished chemotherapy from my first bout with cancer. It hit me like a sledgehammer. I remember being completely stunned and overwhelmed. I was with my husband when the doctor told me, and after a while I said to him, 'Look, let's not think about it right now. Tonight, I'm going to cook us a meal, and then we'll see'. So that day we went to the market to pick up some ingredients and prepare a good meal. I cooked for a long time, and we enjoyed ourselves. Like playing the piano, cooking allows me to concentrate fully on something other than my illness. It brings me pleasure both in the sharing and the joy of doing. Cooking also enabled me to let go!"

Min-Jung Kym

We don't want this book to be interpreted as yet more instructions for patients. It shouldn't be seen as more rules to follow, nor should it appear as a kind of Holy Grail that puts an additional burden on patients when they are already dealing with so much. Once again, we cannot emphasize this enough -- it's normal to be afraid. Nothing about the cancer ordeal is normal. Both doctors and patient alike have to acknowledge this from the start. This is fundamental to overcoming fear and suffering. Start by naming your fears, identifying them, without feeling guilty about having them. Give yourself permission to voice them, to talk about them. If you respect this period of listening to them, feeling them, it then becomes possible to overcome them.

There is no one reproducible model that can be applied to all patients. Each patient is unique, with a particular history, tastes and motivations. Here again, the role of doctors and carers is crucial. Take the time to get to know patients and their specific needs, re-evaluate them often, always talking and listening. These are some of the keys to helping patients put their lives before their illness.

Everyone can find the resources within themselves and their surroundings to remain anchored in life. Regularly cooking, gardening, meditating, seeing friends, exercising or playing sports, reading, working… In reality, everyone has the means to continue living, to create a space outside the illness. No one therapy or activity is better than any other. The right one is the one that suits you as an individual. We encourage patients to pursue their existing hobbies and to take up others, depending on their needs, their desires, their health situation, their place of residence. This means developing coordinated treatment plans in which the carers make themselves available to patient as partners in their daily lives.

Getting access to your rights

Almost anything is possible provided you can get access to it. In the absence of a one-stop shop or establishments offering patients a full range of services, it's often complicated to find your way through the existing systems, to know what's possible according to your physical condition, what's accessible, what isn't... For several years, governments have been conscious of the need to improve patient quality of life and have developed tools that protect patients from being treated unfairly or from being prevented to take part in certain aspects of their daily lives.

This is true in the workplace, for example. While this is obviously not applicable to all cancer patients, some are able to continue their professional activity by adjusting their working hours. Working life can be integral to a person's sense of fulfilment and when possible and desired, it's essential to allow patients to keep working. However, even today, cancer remains an obstacle to accessing or maintaining employment. INCa has shown that 20% of people who had a job at the time of their diagnosis no longer have one five years later.[24]

---

24. "Five years after a cancer diagnosis, quality of life and employment status remain strongly impacted," VICAN-5 collective study, INCa, June 2018.

This led in France to the creation of the "therapeutic part-time" work plan. As the term suggests, this means that continuing to work can be beneficial for patients. In agreement with their healthcare provider and employer, cancer patients can organize a more flexible schedule and keep working part-time. A complement to their part-time salary is provided per day by their health insurance. This makes it possible to stay involved in their workplace or of making a smooth transition back to work after sick leave.

Whether or not you talk about your illness in the workplace is a personal decision, and is in no way an obligation. You can choose voluntarily to share this information, but your employer must keep it confidential. You should decide according to your own conscience, depending on their relationships with your employer and your co-workers. Studies show, however, that when the environment is conducive to sharing your diagnosis, being able to talk about it simply and openly significantly improves the quality of life at work for people with chronic illnesses[25].

Moving, searching for an insurance policy, adapting your home to accommodate your physical condition… patients also need equal access to financial services in order to pursue their goals. Borrowing money can be extremely complex, and many patients still face discrimination as a result of

---

25. "Le parcours de santé des personnes malades chroniques ", guide by the collective (Im)patients, Chroniques et associés, 2019. Downloadable in French at: https://www.endofrance.org/wp-content/uploads/2019/10/guide-parcours-de-sante-despersonnes-malades-chroniques-edition-2019.pdf.

their health status. Even if it's not yet systematic, most cancer centres propose social workers who can help you understand the possibilities and guide you through the process. You should never hesitate to ask for help to enforce your rights. For example, the "right to be forgotten" means that cancer survivors applying for a loan are no longer legally obliged to disclose medical information after a certain period of time. Loans cannot be refused nor can premiums be increased because of their illness.

Apart from these very practical issues, there are also support systems to help patients maintain their leisure activities or even take them up for the first time. In France, if participating in sports isn't possible in the institution where you're being treated, patients can contact the "Maisons Sport-Santé" network. Establishments set up all around the country connect people suffering from long-term illnesses with sports professionals who are specially trained to support patients in keeping with their specific needs. A European social security card can cover your participation in all member countries of the European Union. For young people with cancer who want to travel, being ill no longer means that you can't take a holiday.

II.

Healing body and soul

1.

A patient-centred approach: the Institut Rafaël model

Charles Trenet, *Douce France*: my uniqueness

"I decided to include this song by Charles Trenet on my album *Sounds for the Soul* because I have a very personal relationship with it. This song is an integral part of my story. I'm British, having grown up in London, with South Korean parents, and now I'm also French. *Douce France* is a song that beautifully illustrates my connection with France since moving here.

When I arrived, I was told the best way to learn the language was to read and listen to song lyrics. They are at times complex, but enable you to grasp the soul of a language. Music is intimately linked to the brain's language centre, which makes it a valuable tool for linguistic learning as well as for recovering speech after a stroke. I was delighted to immerse myself in lyrics by Charles Trenet, Boris Vian, Georges Brassens... and so many others!

Douce France is a way for me to affirm my Frenchness. My history with France also includes the history of my illness. I consider myself lucky to have received medical treatment in this country where PET scans are available for all, where my colon cancer was quickly diagnosed and treated. This, too, is what France is.

> There are many possible key arrangements for this song. I play it in F major, a fairly simple and versatile key. It's joyful and light. *Douce France* is another one of my 'Madeleine de Proust'. It brings back memories that remind me of my uniqueness and arouses happy feelings in me."
>
> *Min-Jung Kym*

Respecting the uniqueness of every patient we treat. In this book, we want to show how important it is to consider the patient beyond the illness, to consider every part of the human being. Patients see themselves as whole entities, and this is as it should be. Sometimes you have step away from medicine and think about the individual. To receive and address patients and their suffering, physical or not, and their vulnerabilities, whatever they may be.

At the institute, we practice what is called integrative medicine – medicine that focuses not only on the disease but on the entire person, in order to give patients all possible resources to help them live with their illness and keep moving forward. Not just treating the diseased organ or the physical pain, but helping patients articulate their future goals in spite of their ordeal. This is what we want to achieve.

There is strong demand from patients for support that takes account of all their needs, all their uniqueness. Progress has already been made in this regard; many medical establishments offer complementary care. But for the most part, these institutions only offer this kind of support in order to reduce a treatment's side effects. This left a void, and we wanted to take whatever time was necessary to fill it.

The origins of the Institut Rafaël: the cake lady

"The inspiration behind wanting to establish my own integrative healthcare centre came while I was treating one of my patients, an 85-year-old woman who had always been extremely active and involved with those in her neighbourhood. Every day, she would bake cakes for the students and underprivileged people around her. After her breast cancer diagnosis, she was reluctant to undergo treatment. It just so happened that many years earlier, my grandmother had been a doula and helped women give birth in Morocco. When she heard this, she realised that she'd been delivered by my grandmother! Then and there, she trusted me and agreed to be treated, and gave me permission to take care of her.

Since France is an extraordinary country that offers universal healthcare coverage for everyone, she was able to receive the best, most advanced care to treat her cancer. But after treatment, she stopped baking cakes and refused to leave home.

At the time, I had set up an association called 'Esthètique & Cancer', and I turned to it to try to find a solution. We put together a physiotherapist, a beautician, an osteopath and a psychologist who gave her treatments at home. A month later, she was back outside distributing her cakes.

That's when I realised that I wanted to build an institute that would offer patients personalised support that would help them get back to their lives despite the illness."

Alain Toledano

Cancer is traumatic. It changes the sufferer permanently. Patients obviously need support during their treatment, but they also need it afterwards.

The post-cancer period is long. It takes five years before you are considered to be in remission. During this time, the fear of recurrence hangs over those in remission like the sword of Damocles. This fear does not magically disappear from the patients' lives at the end of this period.

Patients need support in their cancer journey and places where integrative care is available helps them make the transition to the post-cancer period. Patients are given the tools they need to envision life after cancer. In addition, after the accompaniment throughout the illness, care cannot be limited to the time of active treatment. Patients need follow-up care and help managing their side effects and adapting to their new reality. They need support in preparing this step so they can re-appropriate their lives. It is important to enable patients to imagine their post-cancer life and to ask for long-term support that corresponds to the enormous impact the disease has had on them, because life after cancer begins as soon as the cancer is pronounced.

A space dedicated to patients

A personal pathway

"At the very beginning I had an appointment with the treatment coordinator. I was immediately struck by the level of detail involved in defining the kinds of care a patient will receive.

Several thematic questionnaires were used as a basis for in-depth discussion. We talked about my state of mind, my fears, my hopes, what I was looking for in terms of care. We also spoke for a long time about my relationship with my body and about my family and friends, and the type of accompaniment I would need depending on the support I would have elsewhere. Together we analysed all this and defined the treatment I would follow. Since I felt very supported by the people close to me, especially by my husband, it seemed I didn't need much psychological support. On the other hand, it was clear from our discussions that my interest was very focused on food-related issues, so I was signed up for cooking and nutrition workshops. My coordinator and I also discussed the fact that I was used to exercising, and I elected to take part in dance therapy, and she noted that I could be contacted whenever specific sports activities were organised. We then identified a third area of care involving relaxation techniques. Once it has been defined, the treatment plan is re-evaluated several times; it changes constantly in keeping with the way the patient's needs evolve. Although I have finished my cancer treatment, I do not rule out the possibility of seeing a psychologist. While I'm no longer dealing with the disease on a daily basis, the fear of recurrence is increasing. I still have a great deal of support around me, but those close to me are not psychologists. With my proposed treatment plan, I felt as if I was receiving a unique, tailor-made programme built with me and for me, a programme that was not written in stone and that was personalised, not standardised."

Min-Jung Kym

At the Institut Rafaël, the desire is for patients to not feel powerless. We wanted to create a space dedicated entirely to them, one that brought together all the care and support they would need to cope with cancer. You can't separate the disease from the combination of emotional, social, professional, sexual and psychological aspects that make up a patient's life.

On arrival, patients are referred to a coordinator who is responsible for working with them to build a care plan adapted to their needs, developed in a balanced exchange in which the patient's voice has its rightful place. The care they decide upon during the interview can be adapted at any time according to the needs the patients express as time goes on.

The objective is to design a completely personalised care path. Several areas of care are identified according to patients' typical needs: movement-based, nutrition-based, psychological, artistic and socio-professional. More than thirty treatments are offered at the institute, and they are completed with other regular activities, healing circles and partnerships with outside associations.

Depending on the needs identified during the coordination interview, the pathway that is designed will allow patients to navigate between these different activities and approaches, at a level that is determined together – the medical team and patients, sometimes even in conjunction with their entourage. All the therapy treatments take place at the institute, so there is no need to leave to work with other specialists or to participate in activities off the premises. Due to the lack of centralized information, cancer patients often spend a great deal of energy moving around for this, energy that could be better used dealing with the disease. Our concept is to offer patients a kind of "cocoon" where they receive all the care they need in one place.

Dancing for the body and mind

"I love to dance, even though I don't dance very well; musicians are not always the best dancers. They pay too much attention to the music and rhythm, ending up ironically out of rhythm, and feeling inhibited.

Even so, I chose to attend the institute's dance workshop. First, because so many people told me that it was very important to be physically active during treatment. I had already taken yoga and Pilates classes, and I thought a dance exercise class would give me another way to exercise, and also an opportunity to learn something new.

Obviously, the connection to music was not anodine in making my choice. Associating body work with music spoke to me. It also helped me enormously to let go. I was also attracted by the fact that I would be part of a group. I was involved in other individual therapy treatments, like sophrology, but I was feeling a bit anxious about being alone so much. I found a great deal of comfort in the many group activities available to patients."

Min-Jung Kym

Those who are called helpers or caregivers, the family and friends of people with cancer, who support them on a daily basis, are also deeply affected by the disease and may also need emotional support. You can't care for patients without taking into account their relationships with those around them. When patients express the need for it, family and friends can become integrated into the support process. This can be as simple as attending a cooking or art therapy workshop with their children, who sometimes have a hard time understanding the disease, or a couple seeing a psychologist or sex therapist together.

The subject of the patient's personal relationships is inextricably linked and are an integral part of care. It is about weaving connections that will enable patients to get back on their feet. This involves the patients' familial and social environment, but it's also necessary to nurture a care environment that enables the creation of this relational fabric.

Precious connections

"I've always hated the notion of group therapy, like the ones you see in American films when everyone's sitting in a circle. It doesn't appeal at all, and to me, they exude a false sense of intimacy. Despite this, I was keen to the join as many group activities as possible, and I appreciated every minute of the exchanges I had with the other patients.

It's in fact like group therapy that's not group therapy at all! Everything happens in a very natural way. We share a lot between patients, in the workshops of course, but also informally, at the coffee machine or in other situations. You meet people you would never have otherwise met, you talk or listen to strangers with ease. At one of the workshops I attended, I was sitting next to a woman my age. There were only a few of us; on average the other patients are older. We began talking and decided to sign up for some activities together, and little by little we bonded. I recently heard that she's expecting a baby, and I'm thrilled for her.

This is probably also because of the atmosphere in the centre. All the patients listen to each other and there's a real sense of caring. There is no judgement from neither the patients nor the carers. This is precious,

because each patient's situation is unique and each patient needs reassurance.
Of course, we are incredibly fortunate that these workshops and treatments are available for us, but above all, what I remember are the moments of sharing with the other patients. I was full of questions. Being able to exchange with other patients was a crucial factor in the healing process. You see that other people are going through the same thing you are. Sometimes worse, sometimes better, and you feel less different, less alone. It opens your eyes to the disease. It helped me understand better, to reason with myself, not to be overwhelmed by fear and guilt, to put things in perspective".

Min-Jung Kym

Group workshops and group treatments are encouraged. Whether or not you are a fan of group dynamics, in the face of an ordeal like cancer, exchange and sharing are essential. No one should remain isolated when dealing with cancer. Group activities should never be forced, of course, but they should always be encouraged, while still respecting each person's personality and pace. And if possible, in a joyful way.

Faced with an illness that often causes patients to struggle with guilt, to blame themselves and to focus on what they might have done wrong, it's more important than ever to share this experience with others in order to put things in perspective. In short, to be with others in order to be better with yourself.

The challenge of multi-disciplinarity

As we have seen, the importance of supportive care has been recognised by all the participants in the health world, by doctors, associations, the government. Organizations such as the Academic Consortium for Integrative Medicine and Health which more than half of the Academic Institutions in North America belong, exist to encourage global dialogue and exchange. Laws have been passed to facilitate access to supportive care, yet accessing it can still be an uphill battle. As we have seen in previous chapters, complementary care has proved its usefulness, both in terms of the patients' quality of life and of improving their survival rate after cancer.

The make-up workshop: far from frivolous

"I was anxious about going to the make-up workshop. It was at the beginning of my treatment, and it was the first workshop I attended. I knew my body was going to change, but I didn't really know what that would mean concretely, and I didn't dare ask too many questions. But as usual, they did everything possible to make us feel comfortable. The workshop started with a giveaway: full beauty kits, from creams to mascara, for all the participants. It was unexpected, and it built up a feeling of trust and was extremely reassuring. Very quickly, the atmosphere felt more relaxed. It became a moment of exchange, even laughter. We were a small group of about ten women, all at different stages of our illnesses. I hadn't lost my hair yet and everyone told me how lucky I was. Everyone had advice to give. As someone who is used to wearing make-up, thanks to giving concerts onstage, I was able to give advice to women who had never worn make-up before and who had a poor self-image because of their illness. On the other hand, I had a lot of questions about what you can do after losing your eyebrows. Seeing other patients at other stages of the disease put things into perspective for me and helped me understand what I was facing too.

The subject may seem light-hearted but it isn't. Yes, we made jokes. Yes, we talked about lipstick and moisturizers. But essentially, we talked about healing, burns, allergies to treatments, wigs... None of these topics is trivial for anyone going through cancer."

Min-Jung Kym

Treatments can be considered as part of your care plan as soon as they have proven their effectiveness. These include certain so-called "non-conventional" medicines such as Chinese medicine or homeopathy. Chinese medicine considers the human being as an organic whole, making no distinction between body and mind. History even tells us that the patients of Chinese doctors only paid for their consultations when they were not ill! Chinese medicine naturally has its place at the institute. Acupuncture, for example, is the only therapy that can relieve certain side effects, such as hand-foot syndrome.

A number of "unconventional" therapies can be very helpful in dealing with cancer's side effects. Some patients who find the courage to broach the subject of these therapies to their doctors talk about remedies and treatments that can be far-fetched. There is a major risk in not listening to them – the risk that patients will then walk away, even refuse treatment altogether. Conventional or not, many therapies offer true relief for the suffering of cancer patients.

We are constantly conducting research in order to improve our knowledge of cancerology, and of all the topics related to holistic cancer-related medicine. Our goal is an inclusive approach to patient care.

2.

Caring for the person

By the time the cancer has been diagnosed, life has already left its mark on the patient. All come with a unique history, a lifestyle, a culture, beliefs, a set of personal ethics, a relationship to their body, their emotions and life plans. This needs to be considered by doctors dealing with disease: no diagnosis, no illness erases the human being behind it.

Illness affects people profoundly, body and soul, especially cancer. Although it is now largely curable, perceptions of cancer are still strongly equated with a death sentence. Patients have perceptions that are linked to their culture and personal history, giving rise to mental images of their cancer. How you deal with your diagnosis is deeply bound up with these images, on your support system and on the trust you have (or don't); in the medical profession.

Contrary to some countries, the French health care system is extremely generous. Coverage is universal; everyone is entitled to quality care and the most advanced treatments. However, like most Western health systems, it tends to ignore this more personal aspect and focus only on the diseased organ and on medical technology. In this book, we are advocating a shift from disease-centred medicine to a patient-centred, goals-directed care. The first step is not to dissociate patients from the emotions they are experiencing. When you live through a traumatic experience such as cancer, emotions can be repressed and impossible to articulate.

To treat the disease, you must treat the patient and take the patient's feelings into account. Dealing with the patients' emotions influences their engagement in their treatment, their active participation in their own care. It's also valuable in helping patients cope with the treatment and its side effects and to improve their chances of recovery. It ameliorates the patient's state of mind considerably, and in particular can help reduce depression and anxiety.

In this, music offers us invaluable lessons. You don't have to be a musician or a neurologist to observe the emotional power of music. Each of us has experienced first-hand the power of a particular song in an emotional situation, complex or not; the joy of dancing together to a lively tune or the deep, almost visceral emotional charge of Mozart's *Requiem*. All of us have felt this, whether we realize it or not.

Music to heal emotions

The emotional power of music

"Let me control the music of a nation and I care not who makes its laws", Socrates said thousands of years ago. The power of music on our emotions, both individually and collectively, has been thought about for a very long time. Today, companies use music to make consumers want to buy their products. Music is used in the cinema to reinforce a feeling of fear, joy or melancholy. And since the beginning of time, music has been used by mothers to soothe children and help get them to sleep.

When life becomes too painful, people may repress their emotions, bury them deep down inside. They become impossible to articulate and sometimes even inaccessible. In these cases, verbal communication has limitations. Art can help us to break down these barriers, and music in particular is an important means of emotional expression. It has the ability to put us in direct contact with our feelings without the filter of conscious thought, to help us escape the straitjacket of social conditioning. When words are useless, music has the capacity to replace them, to bring out what is hidden or ignored. Whether we feel it deeply or not, we all recognize the emotion conveyed by a piece of music. Music can also trigger powerful emotional memories, even unconscious ones. This makes it an ideal tool for expressing, stimulating, but also healing the feelings we experience, for example, when we have cancer.

Stanley Kubrick, in an interview given years after the release of *2001: A Space Odyssey* in which he tried to explain the film, summarised it perfectly. "There are certain areas of feeling and reality – or unreality or innermost yearning, whatever you want to call it – which are notably inaccessible to words. Music can get into these areas. Painting can get into them. Non-verbal forms of expression can. But words are a terrible straitjacket", he said.

Thanks to the research carried out by neurologists, we now understand more and more about the mechanisms that enable music to influence emotions. We therefore know that listening to certain types of music affect stress levels by lowering cortisol levels in the brain. Music also stimulates the hormones related to positive, happy feelings, boosting the brain's production of serotonin and dopamine, two neurotransmitters linked to pleasure. Both of these physiological phenomena are increasingly well-documented by neuroscientists, as we have seen above. In addition, music stimulates the areas of the brain linked to memory. Your knowledge of music – whether you're a specialist or not – and your experiences with it can be used as a weapon to heighten your emotions.

Brahms, *Intermezzo Op. 117, No. 2:* nostalgia and comfort

"This Intermezzo belongs to a group of works composed by Brahms at the end of his life. He called them the "lullabies of (his) life". Like many of the other pieces he composed during this period, it is very intimate, very introspective and reflects his extreme sensitivity. Brahms no doubt wrote it for his great love, Clara Schumann. It's a piece that channels the soul and brings so much comfort. It reveals a rich inner emotional world and is filled with a multitude of colours, with so many nuances to explore. It is an extraordinarily sensorial experience for pianists to play this piece.

This piece is written in B-flat minor, a key Brahms rarely used that brings a certain fragility to this intermezzo. At the same time, this piece embodies many ambiguities. It's unstable in that it shifts to other keys.

I often compare the melody to sewing. It contains many arpeggios, many harmonic flows interspersed with more sonorous parts and dissonances.
Throughout this piece, Brahms tells his story. Its narration evokes suffering, sadness and his dwindling strength. The colours are often sombre but reveal moments that bring clarity and light on the other side. It is melancholic piece, and expresses nostalgia, but it is also extremely comforting because of the lullaby aspect and lyricism.
I listened continuously to all three Op. 117 Intermezzi, but I had never played them. This piece, in particular, accompanied me throughout my illness. It was a special experience for me to learn and interpret it and to record it on the *Sounds for the Soul* album. It's a piece I adore. Its gentleness reassures me. It has a nostalgic aspect, and it makes me reflect."

Min-Jung Kym

Well-known formulas

In 1892, even before neurological discoveries about the effects of music had been made, Brahms already knew which emotions he wanted to convey through his compositions. Even before anyone had analysed how music evokes emotions or how the famous musical frisson is triggered by listening to a piece of music, composers had a very strong intuition about it.

In the Intermezzo analysed above, for example, Brahms plays with changes in rhythm. He alternates gentle arpeggios with more sonorous moments. This is standard practice, one that can be found in many compositions. So can switching from a major key, which is usually associated with cheerfulness, to a minor key, which is often associated with sadness, the way Mozart does in his *Turkish March.* Changing tempo (accelerating or slowing down), key or tonality are classic, well-known compositional rules that have been used since music's beginnings. Without knowing the causes or the physiological mechanisms at work, musicians have always utilised them knowing full well what effects they would have on their audience.

Many years later, scientists sought to identify the exact reason behind musical frisson. They found that ruptures – sudden variations in tempo, mode and key – are indeed often the cause of the intense emotions we experience while listening to a piece of music.[26]

In fact, music stimulates the auditory cortex, which analyses sounds and creates expectations; memory comes into play afterwards. All of us – whether we are musical connoisseurs or not – have an implicit knowledge of music. This "musical working memory" enables us to unconsciously acquire and retain analytical knowledge of music we have listened to from an early age, enabling the brain to analyse a piece of music and its structure and anticipate what's to come.[27]

---

26. Hervé Platel "Pourquoi la musique nous fait vibrer ?", in E. Bigand (ed.), *Les bienfaits de la musique sur le cerveau* (Paris: Belin, Coll. "Cerveau & Psycho", 2018), pp. 15-26.

27. Barbara Tillman "La musique : un langage universel ?", in E. Bigand (ed.), *Les bienfaits de la musique sur le cerveau* (Paris: Belin, Coll. "Cerveau & Psycho", 2018), pp. 27-47.

This implicit knowledge generates expectations while you're listening to a piece of music, meaning that your brain tries to guess what will happen next. When these expectations are satisfied or even frustrated, they create a sense of pleasure or surprise that evokes our emotions. It's precisely these changes of rhythm, tonality or keys, and the rapidity and frequency with which they are played, that provoke the indescribable emotions we feel when listening to certain pieces of music. This formula has always been used by composers, as we saw in the analysis of Vladimir Cosma's piece. It's also intensified by the memories we associate with a particular piece.

In addition to sudden changes, musicians believe tonalities play a role in conveying emotions to their audience. One of the first people to articulate this was Marc-Antoine Charpentier. In his *Règles de Composition*[28] (rules for composing) in the seventeenth century, this leading figure in French Baroque music classified each key and the emotional effect it aroused. This is the way each key was thought about nearly 400 years ago, as conveyed by researcher Pierre Lemarquis[29] in one of his books:

– C major: cheerful and proud
– C minor: dark and sad
– D minor: grave and devout

28. Théodora Psychoyou, "Les règles de composition par Monsieur Charpentier : statut des sources ", in Catherine Cessac (dir.), *Les manuscrits autographes de Marc-Antoine Charpentier*, Mardaga, coll., "Études du centre de musique baroques de Versailles", 2007, pp. 201-221.

29. Pierre Lemarquis, *Sérénade pour un cerveau musicien* (Paris: Odile Jacob, 2009).

– D major: joyful and very proud
– E-flat major: cruel and harsh
– E-flat minor: terrible, dreadful
– E minor: feminine, amorous and plaintive
– E major: quarrelsome and shrill
– F major: furious and violent
– F minor: dark and plaintive
– G major: sweetly joyful
– G minor: serious and sublime
– A minor: tender and plaintive
– A major: joyful and pastoral
– B-flat major: sublime and joyful
– B-flat minor: dark and terrible
– B minor: lonely and melancholy
– B major: hard and plaintive

Several centuries later, it can be interesting to realise that the way we perceive certain keys has not changed a great deal. Although they of course cannot be regarded as absolute abstract truths, the following are now commonly accepted rules regarding the characteristics of different keys:

– C major: totally pure, expresses innocence and simplicity (Bach's first prelude in C major and Mozart's Aria *Dove sono i bei momenti* are composed in this key)

– C minor: sweetness and solemnity. All the nostalgia and sighs of the heart are embodied in this key

– C-sharp minor (or D-flat minor): lamentation and intimacy. Undoubtedly the most intensely melancholy key, it is used in Beethoven's piano composition *Moonlight Sonata*

– D-flat major: sonorous and rich, a broad key often used for nocturnes

– D major: triumphant, proud and spiritual, often used for symphonies, Alleluias, marches and choirs for religious music

– D minor: melancholy. Often associated with turmoil and anguish (two important pieces were composed in D minor: Mozart's *Piano Concerto No. 20 in D minor, K. 466* and Beethoven's piano sonata *The Tempest*)

– E-flat major: strong and dignified. The key with the greatest expressive variety. Seriousness, solemnity and courage – it embodies them all. The key used by Harold Arlen for *(Somewhere) Over the Rainbow*

– E-flat minor (or D-sharp minor): gloomy and macabre, expresses anguish and the darkest despair. Simply put, the darkness of the soul. If ghosts composed music, they would undoubtedly use this key

– E major: the most luminous key, expresses joy and splendour. Elgar wrote his *Salut d'Amour* in this key

– E minor: sorrow, restlessness of spirit but also a form of naivety. Curiously, a favourite key of guitarists and heavy metal musicians! It is also used in Liszt's *Vallée d'Obermann*

– F major: joy and peace tinged with nostalgia. Used in *Douce France* by Trenet and in *Spiegel im Spiegel* by Arvo Pärt

– F minor: sensitive and melancholy. Sometimes associated with funeral laments

– F-sharp major (or G-flat major): clarity and brilliance in F-sharp major. But in G-flat major, it expresses sweetness and richness, and is the key used in Schubert's *Impromptu No. 3, Op. 90,* included on the album

– F-sharp minor: a ghostly key. Conveys passion but also contains an element of mystery

– G major: gentleness and solace, evokes a feeling of youth. It has a form of simple grace and a luminous, pastoral character. Vladimir Cosma composed *Reality* in G major

– G minor: sadness, but also calm and quiet joy. Evokes a dreamy melancholy and has a sentimental dimension

– A-flat major: sentimental and dreamy, the key Bach chose for his *Arioso*

– A-flat minor: sadness. A-flat minor perfectly depicts the oppressiveness of a heavy heart, and more generally everything linked with the struggle against adversity

– A major: hope and youthful gaiety, almost a declaration of youthful love. The key used in Mozart's *Alla Turca* sonata, which can be heard on *Sounds for the Soul*

– A minor: tenderness

– B-flat major: evoking hope and ambition. An open, clear and luminous key. Composers like it a great deal. Also expresses a form of quiet contemplation

– B-flat minor: quiet expectation and hope. Rarely used. Brahms composed son *Intermezzo Op.117, No.* 2 in this key

– B major: boldness and pride, rarely used.

– B minor: patience, quiet expectation and hope. Evokes calmness and acceptance of fate, like submission to a divine decision

In light of this analysis, we can see that music is a powerful emotional tool. Composers and musicians are aware of this power. Music therapists are conscious of its scope and use it to enable their patients to overcome difficulties and to express or reconnect with their feelings. Thanks to music, an environment conducive to expressing emotions can be created, and certain feelings can also be aroused. In the course of a session, therapists can adapt to what they perceive a patient is feeling and establish through music a dialogue that makes it possible for us to connect with and confront our emotions.

The emotional pulse as a vital constant

An excessive focus on medical technology

For a long time, medicine was essentially spiritual. It focused on spirits, on higher forces, but also on feelings. This is clearly demonstrated in the theory of the four humours developed by Hippocrates, the father of Western medicine. According to this Greek scholar, the body is made up of four basic elements – air, fire, water and earth – which contain four qualities – cold, hot, wet and dry. Air is hot and wet, water is cold and wet, earth is cold and dry, and fire is hot and dry. This theory of the four humours or bodily fluids, which he believed were main causes of disease, was closely related to this theory. The four 'humours' were blood (associated with a sanguine or jovial temperament), phlegm (associated with a phlegmatic or listless temperament), black bile (a melancholic or anxious temperament) and yellow bile (associated with a choleric nature, prone to violence). Illness was said to arise from the emergence of an imbalance between these humours, the elements associated with them and their characteristics.

The school of thought founded by Hippocrates thus presumed that disease is always beyond our control; that it arises from unknown external causes influenced by the seasons, the stages of life, but also by the afflictions of the patient's soul. He placed nature at the heart of the healing process. Hippocrates' thinking has endured for over twenty centuries in Europe. In the eighteenth century, didn't Voltaire state that "the art of medicine consists of amusing the patient, while nature cures the disease"? This approach was often criticised, in particular because of the remedies used to heal the sick, in particular bloodletting, which was much more likely to kill patients than to cure them! A century before Voltaire, Molière had already mocked doctors' ignorance and their dangerous remedies. Although we have moved away from this thanks to all the advances made in medicine, it's important to highlight the fact that Hippocrates' approach never dissociated body and mind, and that he remains a reference in terms of medical ethics.

Little by little, medicine became scientific, and this is a good thing. We learned about the human body, its composition and functioning. We understood the fundamental importance of hygiene. We invented essential treatments that saved the lives of millions of people, as with chemotherapy and radiotherapy. Thanks to research, we are still making tremendous progress, thus making it possible for more and more cancers to be cured.

Along with this progress, however, technology seems increasingly to be taking over the medical field. Over time, it has become organised and divided into more and more specialised specialities and sub-specialities that focus on a specific type of disease or organ. The various departments operate in isolation, disconnected from one another, making it difficult to think collectively and comprehensively about patients as individuals. More often than not, it must be admitted, this is detrimental to caring for them.

Technology gives us feeling we are in total control, but in fact, this is only an illusion. We rely exclusively on technology for decisions we make about patients, very often without the patients being involved. We forget that medicine is above all a human matter, "an art" that "is not and can never be an exact science", as Immanuel Kant said.

While various health system reforms, like cancer programmes, favour more global approaches, they merely reinforce this process. By limiting the time spent with patients and neglecting preventive care – although we know that good prevention policies on risk factors such as alcohol or tobacco could prevent 40% of cancers – public healthcare policies are opting for technological medicine that tends to lose its human face.

Including humanities in medical care

"By nature, my job is technical. It consists of targeting and destroying cancerous cells with rays emitted by an ultramodern machine. That's what radiotherapy is. It would be entirely possible for me to work in a basement and have almost no contact with my patients.

I intentionally chose the opposite. Perhaps it's even the job's extreme technicity that led me to choose a much more human approach. Since the beginning of my career, I have found it hard to bear the pervasiveness of technology and the resulting lack of human contact. It's in my nature to try to understand others, to enjoy my relationship with others.

But it takes real effort to get away from medicine. For the doctor that I am, it's not particularly natural. In a single day, I see an average of thirty patients in consultation. Each patient has a specific story; these are extremely different cancers with complex pathologies, each at a different stage and with specific adapted treatments. I want to cure them all. Faced with the complexity of the disease, technology is a resource. A resource that contains a certain truth – such and such a treatment cures such and such a disease. Nevertheless, we must try to distance ourselves from the theoretical refuge and consider the person we have in front of us. This is the choice I make every day, because it's essential to include the humanities in medical care. I know how useful it is for patients, and how useful in dealing with the disease."

Alain Toledano

Restoring self-awareness

As positive as these scientific advances are, they are no longer enough if we are to fully meet patients' expectations. Even if we choose health establishments or doctors in terms of their professional reputation, we are no longer satisfied by competence alone. The compartmentalisation of various medical specialities can lead patients to fear (often quite rightly) that information does not circulate sufficiently between the various specialists with whom they are dealing, and is therefore preventing coherent care.

Patients expect to be listened to, to dialogue, to be cared for in a way that recognises them as individuals, and that takes into account their specificities, their values and their particular needs, both physiological and emotional. This is particularly true for patients with chronic or complex diseases such as cancer, which require the intervention of several specialists and lead to many side effects.

As shown in previous chapters, cancer does not only affect people's physical health; it also affects their social, sexual and psychological health. A patient's professional life is disrupted, certain life plans may be called into question: projects to have a child, to move, to change jobs... And the lives of those in the patient's entourage, who are often at the forefront, also change completely.

A cancer diagnosis constitutes a veritable trauma that lasts for several years. When you experience trauma, there is a kind of 'disconnect' between body and mind. In a way, this affects your perception and your awareness of yourself. In order to cope, some patients leave their body, in a sense abandoning it to treatments, to medicine, and dissociating it from their mind in an attempt to find a safe haven. The proliferation of carers and medical exams and the depersonalisation of medicine can reinforce this feeling of you becoming lost in the process. Patients can feel ignored, objectified, like numbers in a system that ultimately has nothing to do with them. In the end, they no longer feel like themselves.

Neurologist Pierre Lemarquis[30] considers that music promotes resilience, that it can enable patients to find a new self-awareness. He finds that because of the way it interacts with memory, music makes it possible for us to connect with our memories, our history and our culture. We can then reconnect with the foundations of our sense of self and little by little recover our emotional and relational abilities.

In addition to what music or other non-verbal therapies can offer, doctors and carers in general have an equal part to play in this process. This is even an obligation.

Hippocrates – once again – defined the principles that should guide doctors in their professional practice. When they take their oath, they affirm: "I shall respect all people, their autonomy and their wishes and exercise no discrimination in respect of their social standing or beliefs. I shall take action to protect them if they are weak or vulnerable or if their integrity and dignity are threatened. Even

30. Pierre Lemarquis, *Sérénade pour un cerveau musicien* (Paris: Odile Jacob, 2009).

under duress, I shall not use my knowledge to violate fundamental human rights."

In other words, physicians must take responsibility for their patients' vulnerabilities. Our role is not simply to heal an organ or treat a disease. Caring is the primary mission of healthcare providers. We cannot confine ourselves to a physiological reading of our patients' health status. Health as the search for a state of physical, mental and social well-being – this is now the official definition of health in the constitution of the World Health Organization – and not merely the absence of disease or infirmity. This is the equation we advocate when helping cancer patients. It's important to ensure that patients are able to experience this period fully, without being in denial of their fears, without being disconnected from their bodies, being seen as whole people.

For philosopher Emmanuel Levinas[31], the encounter with "the Other" is from the outset a question of ethics. It places us in a position of responsibility regarding the vulnerabilities of the stranger. "The intersubjective relationship is asymmetrical. In this sense, I am responsible for the Other without waiting for reciprocity, even if it costs me my life," he explains. According to Levinas, the face of the other is in itself a vulnerability, a call for help that you are responsible for as soon as you enter into a relationship with the other.

Everything shows us the value of accompanying patients in a way that takes into account all

---

31. Emmanuel Levinas, *Éthique et infini, dialogues avec Philippe Nemo* (Paris: Fayard, coll. "Sciences Humaines", 1982).

their dimensions as human beings. It's our duty to consider the feelings expressed by patients but in fact, this is also a more efficient way to help their recovery. It's not enough to treat a person's body without taking care of their soul. Medical consultation is by nature an asymmetrical exercise. Just as one takes a patient's blood pressure, one should also take the patient's emotional pulse. Understanding the patient's emotional needs, moods and cognitive biases are the keys to a successful consultation.

Decoding patients' deep-seated feelings enables us to give them a response, to offer them the resources they need to feel better, to live better, to better accept their illness and to better follow their treatments. We can then meet their expectations in terms of care and consideration. The patients' emotional environment is a strategic area for carers. Once we manage to establish a trust relationship, we create the best conditions for patients to create positive mental imagery. Then we can focus on the illness, on the organ, and in this way build an effective treatment framework.

3.

Releasing negative emotions

Before the diagnosis, the cancer already there

"It started with feeling a little lump on my breast. It was very slight, almost nothing, but I felt something was wrong. I went to my gynaecologist, who reassured me and told me to wait and see how it evolved. Three months later, I detected another lump, this time more noticeable.

From then on it was it was a string of appointments with the gynaecologist, mammogram, the biopsy, then more waiting. Three weeks between the initial mammogram that concluded there were micro-calcifications and the results of the biopsy telling me what kind of cells they were. Three weeks of asking myself what would happen next.

Finally, the results came through: there were cancer cells. Again, everything accelerated. An operation to remove the tumour had to be performed quickly. The surgeon thought it was a tumour in situ, meaning the cells were limited to a specific place, that removing the tumour would be enough to stop it from spreading. Since it could be easily treated and cured, it wouldn't be called cancer yet. For me, this was a huge relief. After the operation, everything would be over and I could move on.

But after the lumpectomy, they uttered those three words, 'You have cancer'. The cells were more aggressive than they'd thought, and the cancer had already spread. By then it was mid-July. I had already been operated on, been worried, been reassured. More than four months had passed between the moment when I detected the first signs and the diagnosis. From the beginning, the idea I might have cancer had been on my mind. It took four months to be sure, after weeks of emotional turmoil."

Min-Jung Kym

Going through cancer generates a string of negative emotions that are actually present even before the actual diagnosis is made. Fear of the disease arises at the first, even imperceptible signs. This can sometimes lead people to postpone a doctor's appointment or a screening for fear of facing this anxiety-provoking reality. Although scientific progress is making it possible to cure more and more kinds of cancer, cancer is still overwhelmingly associated with death. Hair loss, weight loss... very visible physical side effects contribute to this image. The point is obviously not to deny the seriousness of a cancer diagnosis, but to show that this collective imagery helps accentuate the fear and anxiety felt by the people confronted with it.

With a view to providing overall, global, person-centred care that takes into account the patient's emotions is an integral part of the process. A disease such as cancer summons essentially negative feelings. Since we know that music has soothing qualities and can act as a natural antidepressant, what can we do about the anger, frustration or despair that can feel overwhelming when you have cancer?

Philosophy and psychology teach us to welcome and accept our darkest thoughts and feelings, and they presuppose that this is the *sine qua non* for overcoming them. But in the context of cancer, this is particularly difficult to accomplish. It's normal to rebel against your condition when faced with a serious illness. It's normal to suffer, to reject what's happening. Accepting your suffering does not mean being in denial. It doesn't mean that the cancer will disappear. Embracing your condition does not mean finding pleasure in it. The first step in such a journey is to recognise what's there, unvarnished, without artifice.

Sadness, anger and anxiety are unpleasant emotions. No one seeks them out. It's not easy to confront them. Yet we've all felt – even if only as teenagers – the paradoxical pleasure and solace you can experience by listening to sad music when you feel unhappy. It's not only gentle, melodious songs that provide relief. Thanks to its cathartic power and its ability to bring out emotions, music has proven itself to be a useful tool in this situation.

A trying journey

Mental health

Long before the first appointment with an oncologist, patients have already had the time to become more fragile mentally. The medical exams, the waiting, often a first surgery... Several weeks, sometimes several months can go by before you know for sure what you're suffering from. This is not because the health system is slow but rather because of the time it takes to establish a reliable diagnosis. From the outset, the medical time frame differs from the patient's time frame. This difference in perception often leads to misunderstandings on both sides, and can intensify an already negative feeling in people waiting for a diagnosis.

Starting with the very first symptoms, you're going down a path that's marked by fear and suffering. A path that can feel even longer than it is. Fear plus the possibility of death and pain have already come into play while doctors are still trying to precisely define the disease the patient is suffering from. All this creates the perfect conditions for mental distress even before the doctor has uttered the word "cancer", even before the disease has been officially diagnosed.

Each medical exam is followed by a wait. Each result brings with it its own set of speculations and Internet searches to try to better understand the meaning of the words and numbers. Starting from the first mammogram – from the very first signs, in fact – the idea of cancer is lurking in a corner of your brain. The dread, the doubts, the anxieties. The inner turmoil begins long before the diagnosis. The disease has already made its mark.

We often associate the stages following a cancer diagnosis with grief. The famous "five stages of grief" – denial, anger, bargaining, depression and acceptance – were identified by Dr. Elisabeth

Kübler-Ross[32] in 1969. Contrary to commonly held belief, these stages are not only experienced by those who have lost a loved one, but by patients with an incurable disease. It's therefore not surprising, even if cancer is not always incurable, that they are frequently seen in people with cancer. It's up to carers to take the time to help identify their patients' emotions in order to provide the best possible response.

But be careful not to get lost by adhering too strictly to this model which, as Elisabeth Kübler-Ross herself indicated, is not an empirical rule but rather an outline of the emotional states people most commonly experience. It cannot be said too often: all patients are unique. They face the disease with their own history, personality, culture and way of dealing with adversity. Applying a theoretical formula to individual experience is always risky, especially when dealing with emotions. It can also create uncertainty in some patients who do not relate to any of these stages and lead to greater confusion.

Betrayed by your own body

Cancer is often experienced as an injustice. It gives rise to an intense feeling of disbelief. Cancer is an extremely guilt-inducing disease. You never stop questioning yourself, feeling ashamed, trying to understand where you have gone wrong. Many

32. Dr. Elisabeth Kübler-Ross, *On Death and Dying* (London: Macmillan, 1969).

patients feel responsible and blame themselves for what is happening to them.

Self-empathy

"'Doctor, why me? What did I do?' This is a question that I'm asked in consultation almost systematically. One of my patients in particular, about ten years ago, could not come to terms with her diagnosis, nor could she get it out of her head that she was somehow responsible for it.

She was in her forties, very health-conscious, very aware of her body. She was physically active and exercised regularly, careful about her diet, and carefully monitored the results of her efforts. She was very gregarious and had an important social life, almost never drank alcohol and didn't smoke. This made her feel that she was in control of what would happen to her body, that she didn't have to worry about so-called 'risk factors'.

In spite of everything, statistics are only statistics, and we can limit the risks but not prevent the disease. Cancer happened to her anyway, as she kept repeating to me during consultations. To help her accept her cancer and stop blaming herself, we had to tell her over and over that it wasn't her fault, that she had done nothing to make it happen.

This is also why we chose to increase the number of opportunities for patients to come together. The diversity of situations and people allows patients to put things into perspective. Understanding and recognising that others aren't responsible for their condition is the first step towards realising that it's also true for you. Through empathy, you can find resources for yourself."

Alain Toledano

Once the diagnosis has been made and treatment has begun, you have to put up with the side effects on a daily basis. The fatigue; days when you can't do anything for more than a few minutes. The dread; stress before each chemotherapy session because you know pain will follow a few days later; and despite all of this, knowing that every week you need to keep going. The discouragement that can set in, and at times the desire to give up. Each consultation, each evaluation gives rise to anxiety and hope, disappointment and euphoria. It's a marathon, an endurance test that you have to go through for several months, one that's physical but also emotional.

You have to relearn how to live with this body that has disappointed you, that hasn't kept its promises, and find the resources within you to hold on, to work at it every day. In the same week, you might feel exhilaration and despair, anger and serenity, joy and sadness. Beyond the physical ordeal, there is also an emotional struggle. Given the difficulty of the journey ahead, the maxim that patients' morale is a determining factor in the ability to heal is far from hollow. On the contrary, it's a very concrete reality.

After four to eight months, treatment comes to a close. But everything doesn't stop. Some cancers require preventive treatments for several years – hormonal treatments after some breast cancers, for example. There is also, as we have already discussed, a long period following treatment before you can be considered officially in remission. You enter a new temporality. It's not about fighting the disease but living life with long-term treatments and side effects and managing the fear. Once the fear of death has been instilled, it's not easy to escape. You become accustomed to a life interrupted by treatments, surgery and doctor's appointments. In spite of everything, this can become a reference point for daily life, a kind of crutch. And then, everything stops. Some patients feel destabilised, a kind of vertigo, when they stop treatment, even though they were wishing for it to end with all their being. They find themselves very alone. A new life begins, but the anxiety doesn't go away.

Expressing emotions in order to overcome them

At this point, how do you manage your feelings? What can you do with the fear, anger or sadness? How can you prevent them taking over, prevent sadness from turning into despair, prevent depression from setting in, and with it impact the disease? There are greater and greater opportunities to let go. We're taught that this ordeal can be transformed into a new stage of life. But concretely, what does it mean to accept your fate, and how do you cope with all these feelings?

Creating space for expression

Releasing anger

"One of the adapted sports workshops available is taught by a boxer. Each participant is given a pair of boxing gloves and set in front of a punching bag. The trainer invites patients to visualise their illness in the punch bag, to unload onto it all their feelings of rage and frustration. There's no limit to the number of punches that can be thrown, the number of words that can be cried out.

Each time, things happen in much the same way. At the beginning, everyone feels a bit out of place, and no one dares throw the first punch. The patients look at each other, a bit shy, as if paralyzed by the magnitude of the task and by this sudden invitation to manifest their explosive anger. It's very rare to be allowed to express anger. Starting in childhood, we are taught to repress our anger and aggression, which are thought of as negative.

And then someone breaks the ice, strikes the first blow, brings out the first scream from deep down in their body. This frees the others, and from then on there's an outpouring of yells, insults, punches against their tumours, their disease. For patients who take part in these sessions, the feeling of release is profound. All of them come out of it drained but glowing with a sense of well-being."

Alain Toledano

Patients are often caught between several, sometimes contradictory injunctions: listen to yourself, hold on despite the difficulties, take time for yourself, rely on your entourage, refocus, remain positive, accept your negative emotions... This list is far from exhaustive. Each of these recommendations is added to an arsenal, a "to-do list" to try to take control of your recovery. After a while, you can get lost in it, and the messages all become blurred. You try to be a good student, to follow all the recommendations people give you. But in reality, it's a mistake to try to control everything.

An emotion is an acute and transient neurophysiological reaction in response to a specific stimulus. It can be positive or negative depending on the context. It's a chronic affective state that can last for several years, composed of numerous emotional or moral elements. Some of these states respond to specific experiences; for example, a patient who comes back for an annual breast cancer check-up will invariably feel the same fear of recurrence. The objective, fact-based results of her mammogram will not change anything; the fear is reactivated at each consultation. In the same way that music can bring back memories and provoke an emotional state, certain events can resurrect emotions and feelings that are sometimes deeply buried.

Guiding patients in their quest for emotional healing requires time on the part of carers and a real understanding of the patient's personality. In order to identify patients' feelings, it's necessary to know them as people. This implies giving them a great deal of space to express themselves.

In order to manage feelings, it's necessary to be able to put a name to them or at least to acknowledge them. This enables us to unleash them. Sometimes for social convenience, sometimes because of an unconscious survival strategy, we tend to suppress negative feelings. We learn to bottle up our anger, to put on a brave face. When emotional pain is too great, the brain finds ways to dissimulate it, to survive. Verbal communication often reaches its limits in this situation. The senses can at times be more useful in releasing repressed feelings, in acknowledging them and thus in overcoming them.

Music as an outlet

Music is a natural vehicle for expressing emotions, positive or negative – sadness, anger, disappointment, even rage can find a powerful outlet in music. Music can also make it possible to confront emotions that have been buried. Researchers have studied the physiological mechanisms at work in music's ability to instil a sense of well-being and calm. We know that music has the power to impose an emotional state, particularly by playing on tonalities, keys and tempo. In addition to "soothing the savage breast", music can evoke sorrow, melancholy, anguish or extreme joy.

Can a piece of music make us feel melancholy or angry? Why do we sometimes need to listen to a particularly sad piece when we are unhappy? Turbulent music does not necessarily make you angry, sad music does not necessarily make you miserable. On the contrary, most of the time, it brings comfort to a tormented mind.

Liszt, *Vallée d'Obermann*: frustration and release

"This piece by Franz Liszt is a very poetic work. It's part of the first of three cycles of *Années de pèlerinage*, which he composed during his travels in Switzerland and Italy. Drawing its inspiration from literature, it's a musical poem, an initiation story. It tells the tale of a young man who travels through the Swiss countryside, a place Liszt idealised thanks to his knowledge of history and poetry. In the course of his wanderings, fascinated by this environment and overwhelmed by the complexities of nature, he asked himself existential questions about the origin of humanity.

This is a piece that resonated with me when I was diagnosed with cancer a second time. I was haunted by the same existential questions as Liszt during his travels. I kept asking myself why this was happening to me. Although I had managed to come to terms with my breast cancer, I couldn't accept my second diagnosis. There was a constant duel in grappling between the frustration and anger of this second cancer and the appeasement of knowing that an early diagnosis made it easily curable.

For me, this piece expresses this feeling perfectly. Liszt described his composition as 'the monochord of the relentless solitude of human pain'. It's extremely powerful and visceral. It expresses the torment, the whirlwind of emotions you can be confronted with, including anger and disillusionment. This piece is not for everyone. It can be very uncomfortable to listen to. From the very first bars, you can feel tension. It's full of dissonance. When I perform it live, members of the audience can have very different reactions. Some love it because it carries them into a fertile imaginary world. Others can be overwhelmed by its anxiety-provoking nature.

The piece begins in E minor, but there are also very melodious parts in E major and it finishes in this key. These movements are very lyrical and soothing. In the midst of torment, Liszt shows us a way out of the darkness.

I used to play it a great deal. It has a very strong introspective dimension; it's a vehicle for confession. During my cancer, I often played the part where it opens up. It becomes grandiose, very sonorous, and gave me an almost physical release. This piece enabled me to transcend my anger."

Min-Jung Kym

This piece by Liszt is characteristic of what are considered "extreme" melodies, which are marked by sounds that are chaotic, heavy and powerful. Extreme music is played *forte* or even *fortissimo* – very loudly. It comprises passages that are full of emotion, general dealing with lyrical themes of anxiety, depression and loneliness. Many people believe this type of music can provoke various forms of anger, a criticism often been made of Wagner. In one of his books, Dan Simmons[33] quotes an excerpt from a letter by Mark Twain during a trip to Europe, when he first saw an opera by the German composer, writing that "a great chorus composed entirely of maniacs would suddenly break forth, and then during two minutes, and sometimes three, I lived over again all that I suffered the time the orphan asylum burned down".

This quotation illustrates perfectly the effect turbulent music can have on listeners. It reinforces an emotion listeners feel at a given moment. In some cases, with people who are deeply depressed, for example, it can increase a sense of uneasiness. Military marches and war songs have been used throughout history to inflame existing hatreds, hatreds that are already extremely present in society. While certain pieces of music can no doubt evoke anger or sadness, it would be wrong to assume that they accentuate only these feelings in their listeners. The situation is far more complex.

33. Dan Simmons, *Lovedeath* (New York, NY: Grand Central Publishing, 1994).

In addition to Wagner, so many composers have created pieces designed to express the torments of the soul, pieces that are beautiful and turbulent, that evoke tears and strong emotions, in no way leaving their listeners indifferent. Chopin, with his *Ballade No. 1 in G minor, Opus 23,* is one example; another is Beethoven with his *Piano Sonata No. 17 in D minor, Opus 31, No. 2,* known as *The Tempest*. Historically, composers have used the key of D minor to depict tragedy and solemnity. Bach's *Toccata and Fugue* is an excellent example of this. It captivates the listener right from the opening passages. Its sonority has a huge impact; it seems to engulf its audience. It's a well-known work that has been used a great deal in popular media and cinema, but also in video games and even telephone ring tones!

It's no accident that requiems by Bruckner, Reger, Fauré and of course Mozart were composed in D minor. In Rob Reiner's film *Spinal Tap,* a mockumentary about a heavy metal band and a monument in American pop culture, Nigel Tufnel, the hero, explains it perfectly while talking about his piece *Lick my Love Pump*. "I'm really influenced by Mozart and Bach…", he says, saying that he's working on a trilogy "in D minor, which is the saddest of all keys, I find. People weep instantly when they hear it, and I don't know why".

One of the pieces that best demonstrates the effect of D minor is probably Rachmaninoff's third piano concerto. "My music is a product of my temperament", said the great Russian-American master, who was known to have experienced periods of depression throughout his life; very few people heard him laugh, and he rarely smiled. What was going through his mind when he wrote this famous piano concerto in this key?

Like Liszt's *Vallée d'Obermann*, all these pieces can be unsettling. They can arouse emotions we generally try to avoid and that we find uncomfortable, yet these are sometimes the pieces of music we go towards despite this fact – or because of it.

This observation has long been noted by philosophers and scientists alike. In reality, listening to supposedly sad music provokes a range of complex but generally positive emotions, from a feeling of calm to a sense of profound beauty. Other studies[34] have shown that people in a sad mood prefer to listen to melancholy or sad music. Liila Taruffi and Stefan Koelsch[35], researchers at the Free University of Berlin, examined the reasons why listening to supposedly sad music can be a pleasurable experience. Their findings demonstrated, for example, that it was appreciated more when participants were experiencing emotional stress or feeling lonely, or when it triggered memories. Their mood at a given moment had a strong influence on their choice of music. Those more prone to empathy or those who are emotionally more unstable were also more likely to derive pleasure from sad music.

---

34. Patrick G. Hunter, E. Glenn Schellenberg and Andrew T. Griffith, "Misery Loves Company: Mood-Congruent Emotional Responding to Music", *Emotion*, Vol. 11, no. 5, 2011, pp. 1068-1072.

35. Liila Taruffi and Stefan Koelsch, "The Paradox of Music-Evoked Sadness: An Online Survey", *PLOS One*, Vol. 9, October 2014.

These two German scientists also showed that supposedly sad music appears to regulate negative moods and provide comfort: the most frequent emotions felt after listening to it were nostalgia, peacefulness and tenderness, thus demonstrating that it can inspire positive emotions. This illustrates that music, even sad, can lead to beneficial effects; it plays a double role, providing both aesthetic pleasure and comfort, and ultimately seems to regulate moods and emotions.

Such studies along with the practice of music therapy suggest that sad music can act as an outlet for negative feelings. It has also been shown that sad songs more frequently incite the famous musical frisson that leads to the release of dopamine. When used appropriately, music can therefore be used to confront negative emotions, via its connection to the archaic brain regions most closely linked to emotions and through its connection to memory, as Mark Twain clearly expressed in his anecdote about Wagner.

Music therapy makes excellent use of these mechanisms to elicit a reaction and engage in a dialogue with patients. It's a valuable tool for dealing with feelings such as anger. Through listening to a melody like the one in Beethoven's *The Tempest*, for example, you can make patients more conscious of the emotions they are experiencing or have buried deep inside. From then on, they have the means to unearth them, express them with a certain detachment, process them, calm them.

Music therapy frequently makes use of improvisation, which stimulates cognitive capacities and spontaneous thoughts. By guiding patients, we can help them connect to powerful emotions like grief, feelings of injustice or shame that may be hidden behind the anger. Sad or turbulent music can then provide ways for them to express the turmoil they are experiencing. At the same time, such music allows patients to face their torment head-on and helps them to distance themselves from it, enabling them to acknowledge and accept it. Like the boxing sessions we mentioned earlier, it offers patients a valuable outlet for the feelings they experience during cancer.

III.

Patients, actors in their own recovery

1.

Empathic music

Music and social bonding

"My radiation therapy sessions, the last phase of my treatment, ended only a few weeks before the first lockdown in France, in March 2020. I fluctuated between relief at having finished the treatments and shock at what was happening in the world.
Of course, I continued to play music at home. For myself, for my family, to get over what was happening to us. But very quickly, I thought about sharing my music with others. So, I opened my windows.
As the music played, one by one, my neighbours started to open their windows. A few more each day. It became a fixture in the day that everyone looked forward to, a ritual in which they listened, and we met through our open windows. We would take the time to chat afte-rwards, to catch up on each other's news. To simply talk to each other.
As the health crisis started to improve, some people would go down and meet in the courtyard of our building. To celebrate the end of lockdown, I performed a 'real' concert from my apartment, with all my neighbours in the courtyard. These were moments of communion. We all felt the same sense of helplessness in the face of the health crisis. Through music, we could be together. Music has the power to help us relate to each other, to come together. During the pandemic, similar situations

took place all over the world. Without music, who knows if we would have shared so much with those who live so near? Would we even have dared?"

Min-Jung Kym

The Italians led the way. In the spring of 2020, when more than half of humanity was forced to stay at home and contact with others was forbidden, music quickly took on great importance. In Bergamo, the first epicentre of the pandemic in Europe, but also in Rome and Milan, Italians went out on their balconies and leaned out of their windows to sing traditional folk tunes, together but at a distance. The empty streets were filled with songs and music. These images were quickly shared around the world, inspiring musicians across the globe. And every evening, as people applauded in unison for the healthcare workers engaged in fighting the pandemic, impromptu concerts were taking place on the street. Songs and melodies played on the violin, piano or guitar wafted through open windows in fragile moments of communion at a time when we could not be one with each other. Bonds were created, feelings of camaraderie were born.

The health crisis that has been affecting us collectively has highlighted the importance of art in our lives, and music in particular. Music provides resources for empathy, the keys to entering into a relationship with others. In addition to being a means of communication, a language, music is also a factor of social cohesion. As such, it offers a number of valuable lessons on human relations, on how to be together, on how to join forces to get through adversity.

In the therapeutic journey of a cancer patient, the care relationship is of capital importance. It conditions the patient's understanding of the illness, their willingness to be involved in the healing process and sense of well-being. This fact tends to be too often ignored by doctors. However, oncologists and attending physicians are key reference points for their patients. The quality of the doctor-patient relationship would benefit from being improved and strengthened. Music is a veritable communication tool with a proven relational dimension that can be useful in building this unique relationship.

Music as a tool for dialogue

Edward Elgar, *Salut d'amour*: a declaration of love

"This track is a dedicated to my husband and my family. Dedicated also to all the families of people with cancer, because they also suffer; their emotions are affected as well.

Cancer is also an ordeal for them. Salut d'amour is like a caress. It acts as a positive remedy for those who hear it. It was written in E major, a key that expresses joy, a key that is very open, very gentle.

Elgar composed this piece for his future wife. It was his engagement gift to her. It's also the gift I wanted to give for my loved ones.

For me, this work characterizes the dimension of empathy that music can take on. Music is a way to send a message, to express feelings to someone, to show them love or gratitude. It expresses this dialogue that we can have through music.

In this work, Elgar conveys profound tenderness for his young fiancée. His love is palpable. The composer's intention here was to express the depth of his emotion. It's truly a declaration of love, one that beautifully describes the intensity of feeling you can have for someone but that also describes the power of human bonding."

Min-Jung Kym

Conveying your feelings through music, expressing your thoughts to others is precisely the effect most composers strive for. Beyond the aesthetic pleasure, beyond a piece's sheer beauty, the musician puts part of his or her soul into it. Just as this "love's greeting" is an affirmation of Elgar's passion for his fiancée, a piece of music can enable us to express and convey our emotions and state of mind. We have already discussed what power music can have on the emotions of the person who listens to it. Immanuel Kant called music "the language of the affects" – perhaps because music most likely appeared before language, and affects are at the heart of the "primitive" or archaic brain, the part of the brain we still have in common with our prehistoric ancestors.

But beyond the specific characteristics of a musical composition, its rhythm, its tonalities, the performer's intention and the manner in which it is interpreted play a significant role in the way the listener hears it. Certainly, the composer's intentions, outlined in the markings and notes on the score, indicate how it should be played, but there is more than one valid interpretation of any given piece of music. As proof of this, the illustrious Austrian conductor Herbert von Karajan showed this time and time again. In his recordings of symphonies by Bach and Beethoven, he presents dozens of interpretations, sometimes radically different, of symphonies by these two great composers.

A performer's mood and state of mind during a concert can have a significant and sometimes an unconscious influence on their interpretation. Musicians don't necessarily play the same piece identically at each performance. Fatigue, hot weather, feelings of happiness or sadness can influence their interpretation, be it via a slightly different rhythm, a gentler touch or a louder volume. A musician might also react to the atmosphere and energy generated by the audience, in a kind of silent connection that is felt by all. Music is never just a solitary pleasure. We interact with music in communion with the performer, the composer and the message the composer wanted to convey.

The American Music Therapy Association defines music therapy as a means of providing avenues for communication that can help those who find it difficult to express themselves in words[36]. A music therapy session is really a wordless conversation between therapist and patient. Therapists use music as a means of communication and expression, as a way of telling the world, or telling yourself, what you aren't able to articulate. Therapists constantly adapt their practice and their choice of music to a patient's reactions. This applies as much to premature babies

36. François-Xavier Vrait, *La musicothérapie* (Paris: PUF, "Que sais-je?" collection, 2018). In English, see https://www.musictherapy.org/about/

in neonatal care as to adults who are capable of verbalising and making their feelings known.

Various tools are available to therapists. Passive listening helps create an atmosphere and generate emotion. Music therapy for newborn babies, for example, is by definition passive, more of a one-way communication with the patient. Nevertheless, its effects are visible from the first days of life. For example, when a calm, gentle piece is played, the heart rate of a premature baby clearly stabilises and calms down, and crying may cease. At this very early age, the cognitive pleasure of listening to a piece of music cannot be a factor in this process. In this situation, music acts as a primitive language that speaks directly to the patient's brain but also to the body; the heart responds to the vibrations of the sound and to the rhythm of the music.

With older patients, there will be more active listening, a more reciprocal exchange between therapist and patient. Several interpretations of the same piece can be proposed, for example, arousing emotions and making patients conscious the emotions expressed through the music. One can also switch to a participatory approach in which the patient plays an instrument or sings. In this case, the relationship is less unilateral, more of a true musical dialogue with the patient.

Whatever means are used – passive listening or active participation – the goal is to establish communication with the patient, to solicit a verbal, emotional or even physical response using music as a tool, enabling patients to express themselves. As soon as a response is obtained, communication is considered to be established. The music therapist constantly adapts to and engages the patient, at times in conversation but often without a word being spoken. In any case, music always plays a central role. Emotions and experiences can be shared in words during a session, but music remains the common language.

Music and empathy

Music is eminently social. Does this mean that it has the power to develop our ability to feel empathy? The term "empathy" was invented by the German philosopher Robert Vischer. He used it to describe the sensibility that leads us to project our emotions onto an aesthetic object. In the eighteenth century, Adam Smith also linked the notion of "sympathy", which is close to our current definition of empathy, to an innate aesthetic appreciation of art, and music in particular.

Even before defining an individual's capacity to understand or feel the emotions experienced by others, like this concept that is expressed through art, art's sensibility and ability to generate collective emotions. Whilst that may not be enough to demonstrate the empathetic virtue of music in itself, it certainly offers some clues.

Music has the ability to induce strong emotions. Extensive studies have been made on music's ability to arouse feelings and to evoke powerful emotional responses through the combined effects of memory and stimulating the parts of the brain associated with emotions. This situates it from the outset as a vehicle for empathy. We are all the more apt to easily understand and feel the emotions of others if we feel connected to our own emotions. The faculty of empathy is developed in particular thanks to the action of mirror neurons, which make it possible to decode facial expressions. This goes beyond what is called Theory of Mind, a cognitive faculty that allows us to anticipate the intentions of others, which is usually acquired around the ages of 4 to 5 years.

The Covid-19 pandemic, humanity's most recent major collective crisis, has also demonstrated the special place of music in our lives. Robert Zatorre, a neuroscientist at the Montreal Neurological Institute at McGill University, coordinated an international study[37] of 1,200 people in the United States, Spain, Italy and Canada, exploring the activities that helped them cope during the lockdown. His results are quite revealing. Music-related activities were the most popular (14.48%), followed by talking with friends, family or colleagues (14.07%) and exercise (12.93%). His results also show that these three activities were undertaken much more frequently than cooking, which came next with 10.79%, and percentages for the 37 other activities proposed in the questionnaire were significantly lower. By demonstrating the links between the musical frisson and the release of dopamine, he showed that listening to music is connected to pleasure, even in times of great emotional stress.

---

37. Herrero, E. M., Singer, N., Ferreri, L., McPhee, M., Zatorre, R., & Ripolles, P. (2020, December 22). *Rock 'n' Roll but not Sex or Drugs: Music is negatively correlated to depressive symptoms during the COVID-19 pandemic via reward-related mechanisms.* <https://doi.org/10.31234/osf.io/x5upn>.

The more his interview subjects were affected by the pandemic because of losing a loved one or a job, or because they were suffering from the effects of the disease, the more likely they were to listen to or play music.

During several months when almost the entire planet was deprived of normal social interactions, a vast majority of people turned to music. In addition to the emotional support provided by music, whose origins have already been explored here, music represented the only prospect of contact with the another. Research by the sociologist Anne-Marie Green[38], who has made a great deal of research on people's relationship with music at different ages, showed that music is above all a "presence" for the elderly.

The empathic dimension of art, and music in particular, is also due to the fact that it responds to a vital need to connect with others, which is also at the very origin of our capacity for empathy. The faculty of empathy originates in the bonds infants need to develop. This is called the need for attachment. This bond enables the baby to enter into a relationship with another person and to learn to distinguish the emotions felt by another person. This need to relate, to be connected to others, follows us throughout our lives. It's as important for our health as our basic physiological needs (eating, sleeping…).

---

38. Anne-Marie Green, *Les personnes âgées et la musique*, Issy-les-Moulineaux, EAP, 1993.

In a recent book, researchers Barbara Tillmann and Emmanuel Bigand[39] conclude that music is a tool for social cohesion; they observed in particular the impact of music on older people with Alzheimer's disease, even at an advanced stage, and the crucial role it plays in maintaining relationships with others. What is no longer possible with speech or memory becomes possible with music, just as babies engage with the lullabies played for them by soothing themselves with music. Music has the power to bring us into a collaborative relationship with the other.

For these two cognitive scientists, the strong need for music that manifested itself during the health crisis can be explained by music's ability to meet the need for social bonding. At a time when contact with others was not permitted, sound became our only means of communication. The need to establish social relationships was expressed through sound, through music. When you synchronise with someone, especially through music, you change your empathic relationship with that person, which immediately seems more pleasant. If everyone gets into the same rhythm, it becomes possible to enter into a collaboration. Music, through the emotions it arouses and the simultaneous aesthetic pleasure it generates, makes it possible to enter into this much-needed collaborative relationship. It thus develops our capacity for empathy.

---

39. Barbara Tillmann and Emmanuel Bigand, *La symphonie neuronale* (Paris: Humen Sciences, coll. "Société", 2020).

A utopian community

This is the utopia Daniel Barenboim, the Argentine-Israeli pianist and conductor, wanted to create. When he founded the West-Eastern Divan Orchestra with the late American-Palestinian scholar Edward W. Said, he was capitalising on music's capacity to create a feeling of empathy. In 1999, the two men decided to create an orchestra composed of an equal number of Israeli musicians and Arab musicians from the surrounding territories (Syrians, Lebanese, Egyptians, Jordanians and Palestinians). Their goal was to promote a dialogue, working for peace between Jews and Arabs in the region. The project was founded on the belief that there was no military solution to the conflicts that plague the Middle East and that the destinies of these peoples are inextricably linked. Since then, the members of the orchestra come together every summer for a workshop lasting several weeks, first in Berlin and now in Seville, and tour internationally once the workshop has finished. From the outset, Daniel Barenboim and Edward Said's intention was to have the orchestra play in every country in the region most affected by the conflicts. In reality, the "Divan" was only able to accomplish this once, in an historic performance held in Ramallah in Palestine in 2005. Today, it's impossible for them to perform in most of the countries represented by its musicians.

After twenty-two years of existence, the conductor acknowledges that this foundational utopia has not been fully realised. But if the West-Eastern Divan Orchestra was not quite able to achieve its hoped-for peace mission, it's nonetheless a beautiful illustration of the fact that a collaborative relationship between peoples in conflict is still possible, at least within the orchestra. Every year for the past twenty-two years, Jewish and Arab musicians have been making music together and performing around the world. Vocations and careers have blossomed, and its members have transcended their situation.

Art in general, and music in particular, frequently appears to be a means of achieving concordance. As Emmanuel Bigand has shown, sharing the same emotion or a moment of aesthetic pleasure with others changes our perception of them and our ability to embrace their feelings. The development of world music, for example, has opened up new horizons for Westerners and provided them with a way, among others, to immerse themselves in and better understand cultures that *a priori* are foreign to them. This is also the thesis proposed by Eric Clarke, Tia DeNora and Jonna Vuoskoski[40]. These professors believe that music helps to create a feeling of collective communion and promotes intercultural understanding. In their study, they quote the English musicologist Nicholas Cook, who in his 1998 book stated, "If both music and musicology are ways of creating meaning rather than just of representing it, then music can be seen as a means of gaining precisely the kind of insight into the cultural or

---

40. 46. Eric Clarke, Tia DeNora and Jonna Vuoskoski, "Music, empathy and cultural understanding", *Physics of Life Review*, Vol. 15, Dec. 2015, pp. 61-88.

historical and not a pessimistic musicology, like solipsism, which proclaims that is impossible."

This is one of the greatest powers of music – to evoke a common emotional state in a large number of people. Isn't it said that a crowd 'vibrates in unison' at a concert or when they hear people singing in stadiums? This brings us back to Adam Smith and his conception of sympathy, the premise of the notion of empathy, which he considered to be "based on a harmonic chord which is not played in unison, but rather set in the resonance of a shared affect[41]".

There are few "universals" in music. The pleasure we derive from it is linked to our cognitive evolution. But the fact remains that while not all populations necessarily have a word for it, music is present, in one form or another, in every country in the world. And for everyone, music is a marker of collective life. Music produces a powerful sense of belonging. This is particularly true in adolescence, when people are forging their identities, questioning their relationships with others and developing a sense of autonomy. Sociologist Anne-Marie Green[42] has shown that music gives adolescents a strong sense of identification with their peers. In her study, she also demonstrates that music participates in the socialisation process by engendering social relationships, relationships we choose freely, unlike our family relationships.

41. Jean-Louis Le Run, " Intersubjectivité et empathie : les miroirs, la musique et la danse", *Enfances et Psy*, 2014/1, n° 64, pp. 16-28.

42. Anne-Marie Green, "Les comportements musicaux des adolescents", *InHarmoniques*, n° 2, 1987.

Thanks largely to its connection to memory, music plays an important role in building a shared culture. The great moments in our collective history, the rituals that punctuate human lives, most of life's foundational events are invariably associated with music. Hymns, lullabies, wedding songs, requiems, ritual dances, even pop culture reinforce our sense of belonging to a collective culture, of being part of a group of people connected by a history and a commonality. In times of crisis or adversity (as was the case during lockdown), we turn more spontaneously to well-known songs, popular tunes or works that have marked our history. In this way, we seek out the emotions and memories these pieces convey. Music thus plays a role in reassuring us and building our identity. It reinforces both the feeling of being oneself and the sense of being part of a collective.

2.

Readjusting the patient-doctor relationship

There are two people in the care relationship. The strength of what we create over time is the patient-doctor bond, and in it lies the power of the interaction and connection between carer and patient. The unique rapport between doctor and patient has undergone major changes, moving over time from an act of charity to an exercise in shared information. Despite this, it remains circumscribed by a great deal of ambivalence. Trust is the essential ingredient, yet a trusting relationship is not always customary. Recent developments in medicine have tended to make it more egalitarian, yet a feeling of mistrust still persists. Some people sometimes see this relationship as a battle.

Despite the positive developments, the medical world is still structurally "violent" in the way it treats people. Care providers can be flawed. They want to transmit simple information and adhere to it, to drape themselves in an absolute scientific truth, but the way in which this truth is conveyed can be brutal. In medicine, there is no culture of transmission, and this can be detrimental to patients. Medicine has not yet invested enough in the way it approaches the relationship between the medical professional and the patient.

Medical consultation is a delicate art, an art made of contradictions, a fragile equilibrium. Finding the right balance between distance and empathy is not easy. But in a care process as dense and complex as that of a cancer, this is crucial. The patient's ability to cope with his or her treatment and illness depends on this delicate balance. Creating this bond requires time and availability to others – two commodities that are too rare in medicine today.

Towards a new equilibrium

A more egalitarian relationship

For centuries, medicine was an act of charity. Intrinsically linked to a spiritual dimension, it was practiced by clerics who cared for the suffering and the needy in charitable almshouses. The poor and the sick were taken in without distinction. At the time, they provided "care" as opposed to "medicine" in the sense that is understood today. The hospital as we now know it did not yet exist. Medicine was already being practised there, but it was mainly a place for curing souls.

In 1656, under King Louis XIV of France, the Hôpital général de Paris—the forerunner of what we now know as hospitals – was created. Its establishment was accompanied by the implementation of a policy in which health issues took precedence over care related to a patient's social and spiritual dimension. This was the beginning of the secularisation of medicine, a process that continued to evolve as science and medical knowledge progressed.

Little by little, medicine developed; knowledge, information and cognizance formed the foundations of medical authority, in direct contrast to patients' ignorance of their illness and treatment. The relation ship between doctor and patient was based on something asymmetrical, hierarchical, often described as paternalistic. The doctor was validated thanks to knowledge, and had all the power over patients, who were passive and totally uninformed about the illness that was affecting them. This logic prevailed until very recently; the basis of the relationship between carers and patients has therefore long been based on a major power differential. As the French philosopher Jean-Philippe Pierron[43] puts it, "medical authority believes its legitimacy is based on the knowledge of some and the ignorance of others". Doctors' legitimacy is thus experienced as authority based on purely scientific and unimpeachable facts.

This imbalanced, top-to-bottom relationship persisted until very recently, but since the end of the twentieth century, this trend has tended to be inverted and two major movements have contributed to this. Scientific progress has meant that many once deadly diseases have become chronic, creating a population of long-term patients who are necessarily taking a more active role in their own care. At the same time, the massification of schooling and

43. Jean-Philippe Pierron, "Une nouvelle figure du patient ? Les transformations contemporaines de la relation de soins", *Sciences sociales et santé*, Vol. 25, 2007/2, John Libbey Eurotext, pp. 43-66.

mostly the development of the Internet has given a much wider public access to medical information and a better understanding of medical issues, greatly accelerating the rebalancing process and profoundly changed the nature of the carer-patient relationship.

However, traces of this top-down relationship remain. Some carers are tempted to see this rebalancing as a power grab by patients, challenging their competence and their legitimacy. They are reluctant to acknowledge their patients' questions. This can sometimes lead to major misunderstandings – and tensions – between doctor and patient.

When lack of trust hinders dialogue

"Before my lumpectomy, I made my own research. Research on the internet can sometimes provoke anxiety, but it can also be useful. I'm a rational person, so I manage not to be overwhelmed by the alarmist information you can find there. I just look at the facts. I read that you can determine the aggressiveness of cancer cells by doing what's called a sentinel node biopsy. The first lymph nodes in the armpit, the ones closest to the tumour, are analysed to see if they also contain cancer cells. So I asked the surgeon who was to operate on me about it.

Right away, I could sense her irritation. She cut me off, reassuring me that it wouldn't be necessary. Refusing to evoke the cancer risk, she seemed to be worried about frightening me, as if hoping to rein in what she perceived as unreasonable anxiety on my part, but in fact, this was completely irrelevant and did not correspond to my state of mind.

A couple of weeks after the operation, with what should have been a simple report of the results turned into a cancer consultation. The tumour was indeed invasive, meaning cancer cells had infiltrated the surrounding tissue.

By the end of the consultation, the diagnosis came like a punch in the solar plexus, even if before I had already felt ready for it. By refusing to talk to me about it, by silencing my simple questions so as not to be alarmist, the doctor had the opposite effect."

Min-Jung Kym

In France, the real turning point in rebalancing the relationship between carers and patients came in the early 2000s, which became legally protected in a 2002 law on patients' rights[44] affirming the need to do everything possible to improve the patient's quality of life during illness. This law validated the rather recent developments by recognising the place of patients in the care relationship and by granting them a certain number of rights within the framework of that relationship – the right to professional secrecy, to dignity, to non-discrimination, but also the right to information and the right to express their wishes.

Remaining challenges

This has led to a new concept of patients, who are better informed, with enforceable rights, as 'consumers'. They are wary of patients and see them to be retaliatory, quick to litigate the relationship and

44. Law n° 2002-303 of 4 March 2002 on patients' rights and the quality of the health system.

challenge decisions made by medical authorities. This also contributes to strained relationships in a context where public health policies, while recognising that patients have a status and a place in the health system, still prioritise medical techniques to the detriment of the carers' primary mission: *caring* for the patient[45].

The ever-increasing technicity, ultra-specialisation and division of each category of medical professionals is multiplying the number of interlocutors for patients with chronic diseases. This is particularly true for cancer patients. Each stage of the treatment process islinked each time through contact with a different person: radiologist, oncologist, surgeon specialising in the organ being treated, surgeon specialising in reconstruction…. Paradoxically, this weakens the care relationship. Patients are often deprived of a privileged referent with whom they can develop the trust essential to the smooth management of their care.

In a way, for patients this leads to a loss of reference points and meaning, contributing to a certain mistrust of the health system. If all participants follow one another without discovering and knowing each other, without working together, if patients are no more than anonymous links in a chain, they may feel they are simply an object of treatment that is purely technical, often impersonal.

We do not always invest the time needed to building the care relationship – the essential cog

45. Jacques Dubin, "La place du patient", *Esprit*, n° 2007/1, January 2007, pp. 40-51.

in the wheel that enables us to weave the singular link between doctor and patient. Many doctors still prefer imaging, technique, and medical gestures. The consultation, the act of taking the patient's emotional pulse, is not considered valuable, either medically or financially. This means a great deal.

At the same time patients – more informed, aware of their rights, often eager to feel they are on an equal footing – are becoming more demanding, trying to assert themselves in a relationship they feel is one-sided.

The persistent asymmetry of the relationship is also, and perhaps above all, due to the fact that it's essential is to accept and accommodate the vulnerability of the other. This is the doctor's duty, the profession's uniqueness: the doctor is there to receive the patient's distress. Paradoxically, this is the aspect in which doctors are least trained. We do not learn how to welcome suffering, how to listen to it and accept it. We are taught more about the distance we need to keep from patients in order to treat them objectively, unemotionally. But we do not learn to face our own vulnerability. Patients are vulnerable, in a position of weakness. No matter how demanding they may be, they tend to idealise medical professionals as tutelary figures and sometimes don't dare to articulate their questions and doubts. The doctor's scientific aura continues to be intimidating. Patients want to please them, to be "good patients", so long as there is a tangible reality behind this expression.

Let's once and for all abandon this relationship between all-knowing authority and ignorant consumer which harms us all, and devote the time needed to address the patient's suffering. The care relationship is neither a battle nor a confrontation. It's built together, as partners, in harmony and mutual respect. Because while the doctor has technical expertise regarding the disease from which a patient is suffering, the patient has experiential knowledge that should be equally respected, because it enables better care.

Finding harmony

Giving voice to patients

Feeling heard

"The circumstances surrounding my cancer screening are a bit particular, but they're pretty common with regard to how hard it can be for patients to express their feelings to doctors. I was young. I had no risk factors and no family history of breast cancer, so I didn't fall into any specific screening category. I routinely self-examined but nothing else, and I really had no reason to worry that I might have cancer. I just didn't think it could happen to me.

But in addition to the small lump I'd found and that prompted me to consult my gynaecologist, deep inside I sensed something was wrong. When I tried to articulate this feeling to my doctor, she reassured me and immediately brushed aside my hypotheses and my doubts. She left no room to discuss my intuition, the feeling, however palpable, that was nagging at me, and I let myself be persuaded to wait a few more months. But deep down, I was still convinced something was there. Three months later, I went back because I had felt another lump, more definite this time, and they started screening tests. In the end, the cancer growing inside me had nothing to do with either lump I'd discovered during my self-checks, but my intuition had been well founded. The cancer that was affecting me was progressing very quickly and very aggressively. I was very lucky to be treated right away: appointments obtained thanks to last minute cancellations and those around me quickly referring me to the right people... But if I had really, fully, been heard from the start, how much time might I have saved in getting my diagnosis? How many weeks of anxiety might have been avoided?"

Min-Jung Kym

Doctors sometimes tend to forget that the body they treat is connected to a human being. When we say that patients have an experiential knowledge of their illness, this corresponds to a very concrete reality. They feel it in their flesh. The pain they articulate is not imagined, even if it does not fit into the habitual canon of symptoms listed in medical textbooks or scientific studies.

Many diseases have only been researched in depth thanks to patients' tenacity. One example is endometriosis, which until very recently was treated very lightly by the medical community. Medical knowledge is evolving. It's not static, and this perpetual evolution is in fact the beauty of science. The three thousand scientific articles published each day on the PubMed search engine should be a source of humility. Doctors' scientific knowledge is by no means the only thing they have to offer. Their ability to understand, listen to and care for their patients is just as important. Without mastering the emotional workings of the relationship, the power of science alone is nothing.

This is actually one of the first requests patients make – not to feel infantilised, to have their suffering fully heard and acknowledged by health professionals[46]. An American study in 1999 suggested that doctors interrupt their patients after only 23 seconds. Where are we with this today? We don't really know, but what we *do* know is that patients are pushing for genuine attention and consideration.

The time spent listening to the symptoms patients describe is essential. Here again, only the patient has knowledge of them. Only the patient is experiencing them. Don't cut things short because a particular word suggests a diagnosis can be made; let the patient finish the telling. This is what can enable you to really understand the illness that is affecting the patient. Allowing patients to express their feelings about their illness, taking the time to let them express themselves provides valuable information for building an appropriate care plan. It's indispensable to value this time spent with the patient. Today, this time spent is not sufficiently considered in terms of the expenses linked with an illness, as if it were not part of the medical action.

Taking the patient's word into account means recognising him or her as a human being. This is a fundamental issue in the care relationship. Making

46. Marco Vannotti, "L'empathie dans la relation médecin patient", De Boeck Supérieur, *Cahiers critiques de thérapie familiale et de pratiques de réseaux*, n° 29, 2002, pp. 213-237.

sure patients do not feel objectified, that they don't feel they are a 'thing', just a target of the medical care. This means they can also have a positive attitude about themselves. You cannot have self-respect if you are deprived of all social recognition.

Listening is also an indispensable tool for relieving suffering. Giving patients the space to express their pain and fears in an unvarnished, non-judgmental way, gives them the consideration they deserve. In a way, listening to them is already treating them. Providing a space for the suffering helps to alleviate it. The emotional part of the suffering is assuaged. Once it's named and understood, it can be accepted more easily.

In the medical consultation, a dynamic of sharing should predominate. We need to try to build an equitable relationship between two human beings; then we can speak of shared information and grant the patient the right to information as expressed in the 2002 law. Because we're talking about a reciprocal exchange of data, from patient to doctor and from doctor to patient. Both partners should be transparent, sincere and truthful. In order for patients to feel authorized to give doctors such information, we need to establish relationships based on trust.

Empathy in the healthcare relationship

Medicine has not sanctified sensitivity, yet it's essential in this eminently human field. This is in fact an established expression. We speak of medicine with a "human" face, or of a "human" doctor to describe a practitioner who seems to have the qualities of listening and empathy. It's necessary to put empathy into the care relationship. Here again, there's a fine balance to be struck. Patients aren't asking to be mothered; they want to be treated humanely and fully considered as individuals.

However, care should be taken not to confuse empathy with compassion. It's no longer desirable to rediscover the compassionate logic of charity that prevailed until the twentieth century, this singular colloquy bringing doctor and patient together. Nor is it a question of suffering with the patient. This would prevent doctors from making and proposing to the necessary decisions with the needed discernment.

It means paying attention to the emotions expressed by patients in consultation, verbally or not. Sometimes, out of a desire to be reassuring, doctors unwittingly minimise the negative emotions their patients express as a matter of social convention. For this reason, real work on doctors' emotions has to be undertaken. This is a prerequisite for building a solid bond between the relationship's two protagonists.

The care relationship is a process in which the carer is involved with the patient. The care relationship is an encounter between two entities. For this encounter to take place, the attention given to the patient should be unmitigated, building a path together, gradually, in response to the feelings expressed by the patient. Better still, by trying to unearth them, understand them, respond to them. The consultation is a place for exchange that should be totally free and without judgement. The resulting journey is carried out by two people, defined by two people, even if it's the patient who will undergo treatment. This presupposes a trust relationship that goes both ways, and doctors need to work towards earning the patient's trust.

Arvo Pärt, *Spiegel im Spiegel*: hypnotic

"*Spiegel im Spiegel* is a very special piece. It's one of the Estonian composer's best known works. It consists of just three notes, delicately repeated in a series of melodic variations that recur in turn. His most important musical and cultural influences, which are drawn from Gregorian chants and his Orthodox faith, can clearly be seen in this piece. He himself defined his musical style as 'tintinnabulant' (like the tinkling of a bell) when describing his minimalist, meditative compositions.

The title, 'Mirror in mirror', is quite self-explanatory: an image that repeats itself endlessly. Arvo Pärt wanted to depict infinity in this composition, and a reason why perhaps it is very often used as the soundtrack for films about space or the universe, such as *Gravity*.

The three notes are reminiscent of Beethoven's *Moonlight Sonata*. The piece is very slow, a bit melancholy and infinitely nostalgic. But above all, the mood is completely serene, completely even. This sense of stability makes it particularly soothing. It feels dreamlike and has the power to transport us to a totally different universe, to another dimension. The emotions evoked by this work come from the introspection and calm that emanate from it, in contrast to our noisy, frenetic world. The performer must have faith in the music, let it speak for itself.

The consistency of the rhythm and notes creates a reassuring framework and catches our attention through repetition. This piece can be described as hypnotic. It's very useful in music therapy. This kind of rhythm can help capture a patient's attention at the beginning of a session, get the patient to concentrate, the way the rhythm of a hypnotist's voice puts you into a hypnotic trance. It enables the patient to feel reassured, to be completely in the moment. This composition illustrates this effect perfectly."

Min-Jung Kym

Music is temporal. It takes time to play music, to listen to it, to experience it fully. But perhaps one of the most intense aspects of the way music affects us and raises our consciousness is how we invest the space where we live, how we live and move in that space. John Cage's *4'33,* a composition that is completely silent, is a striking example of this. The environment we find ourselves in when we listen to it takes on a life of its own: the sounds of a hospital, the quiet of a country house, the car horns on a nearby street.... Listeners create their own music in keeping with their environment. All this affects the way we hear and keeps us present in what surrounds us. A rhythmic constancy as unwavering as that of *Spiegel im Spiegel* also offers listeners space and time.

Music therapists have their own formulas for entering into a symbiotic relationship with patients, for creating the empathetic relationship that allows them express their feelings. Music is particularly useful for entering into a relationship with the other. If we sense agitation in patients or in young children who have a hard time concentrating, we try to find music that can be described as "hypnotic". We can then play on rhythms that will be rather steady. But you still need a musical hook; a piece that is too soft, too hazy, simply pretty or pleasant will not be enough. You need a musical anchor to create a bond with the patient. Music offers an escape and enables patients to express their feelings, allowing them to overcome the agitation they are experiencing. It helps us connect with patients and their emotions, to engage in the "musical dialogue" that takes place in a music therapy session.

Music is one tool for empathy, but others exist as well. In general, in order to be able to discern a patient's feelings, it's essential to pay attention to non-verbal signs. A blinking eye, looking away, blushing, swallowing, a person's mood are all signs that offer information about the person's emotional state. Mirror neurons normally do the rest. They allow us to interpret these signs and adapt our response, to understand what the other person is feeling. The therapist has to be sensitive to these signs and use them, to pay attention to the patient's subtlest emotional expressions, to notice every clue, because very often negative feelings are hidden. You have to pass through the unspoken and explore the patient's emotions before the medicine itself can be involved.

A physical posture, a bodily attitude, a change in one's tone of voice can be enough to create a reassuring environment for the patient. You can work on your gaze to give space to the other person, to their unique character. The role of silence in this context is far from neutral. Silence touches the sensitive being and leaves room for the unspoken. Combined with a benevolent and attentive gaze, it creates trust. The objective is to create the conditions for a calm and honest dialogue.

There is an art to conducting an interview, an art in rhetoric. It's said that words serve to please, move or convince. The rhythm of a consultation can be built around this objective. We can allow ourselves to slow down, to catch the patient's eye and to bring the patient along with us. To help move beyond the feeling of shock linked to the disease and gradually return to the patient's temporality, to accompany them as they move towards treatment. The medical consultation is an exercise in active listening in which the carer should be able to respond, to give something back to the patient.

Medical truth is not necessarily human truth, or, quite simply, the patient's truth at the moment when you're working together. You have to manage to make the two coincide, to take a step back from the medicine. The important thing is to access the patients' capacity to hear, then to accompany them. To be sensitive in the context of the care relationship without diminishing or overprotecting the patient, without overestimating or minimising the patient's distress: simply listening.

3.

Co-creating the treatment plan

Having the means to make choices

"After the somewhat clumsy announcement of my cancer diagnosis, I had to choose an oncologist. I first went to see the one recommended by the surgeon who had removed the tumour. For the first time, I found myself with someone who was not avoiding the issue. The doctor was very frank, which I appreciated. I finally felt I had the full picture. But he also seemed pushy and didn't explain much about the steps of the treatment: When would my breast be removed? Why? I didn't really get any answers to my questions, just a sense of the urgency of the treatment, which I didn't need to be convinced of because I was determined to do whatever was necessary.

I don't particularly need to be pampered, but I do need to understand what's happening to me. These were big decisions and I wanted to feel accompanied, to know what was going to happen, to be aware of what it would mean.

That's when I turned to Alain. I went to see one of his associates who was a chemotherapy specialist, then saw Alain when he came back from his summer break. In the end, working with Alain and his institute suited me best. There was no more aggressive rhetoric but rather a constructive dialogue with explanations. I understood it was better to have the mastectomy before chemotherapy started in order to get a precise idea of how much the cancer had spread. All the care options available to me given my situation were presented clearly. At no time did I feel my hand was being forced. On the contrary – I had the impression they were looking with me for the best solutions in light of my disease's specificities. I was fully involved in the medical decisions being made. As a result, I was able to take ownership of my treatment. I understood the reasons for it, its advantages. I was no longer a spectator, but a participant in my own care".

Min-Jung Kym

The care relationship is built by two people, but so is the care pathway. Although there are fairly standardised care protocols for each cancer, and there are treatments that are indispensable for treating cancer, the fact remains that patients should be involved in the medical decisions that concern them. This is even a right recognised by law. It's also the only way for patients to take ownership of their treatment. Understanding the reasons for it is what allows them to support it and take an active role in it; in other words, to play an important role in it, to be key actors in their own recovery.

The care relationship has evolved a great deal in recent years, and patients have become no longer just the object but the subject. However, the ultimate aim of the care relationship, particularly in the case of chronic diseases and cancer especially, is still to establish a care plan. The patient should also play an active and not passive role in this. This is what the relationship between doctor and patient should lead to. It's important to ensure that the patient not feel objectified by the treatments and medical gestures necessary for recovery, that they feel like a partner in it, completely engaged in their own health.

Announcing the cancer diagnosis, a marker in the care pathway

Announcing the diagnosis is the first stage of care, when the diagnosis is made and a course of treatment is proposed. Treatment begins with words, with the way the doctor addresses and considers the patient. The establishment of trust depends on this. It determines, for a time at least, a patient's ability to make the projection into possible cure, to accept to live in the present.

The importance of the diagnosis announcement was recognized after the first general meeting of cancer patients. The vast majority of patients reported the deleterious effect of their diagnosis and the lack of humanity in the carers' words. Sometimes the announcement amounted to a mere telephone call made between appointments to pronounce the unimaginable: the patient had been diagnosed with a potentially lethal disease. Others were not even this lucky, simply receiving a simple letter – the results of a biopsy, a scan or ultrasound, and the resulting cancer diagnosis. Not one doctor took the time to explain the details of these results, what they meant and how they could be treated.

A few years later, in 2003, the first Cancer Plan in Europe institutionalised a protocol for the diagnosis announcement and defined the phases of explanation and discussion that are included. The announcement has now become the first vector of information and involvement for patients[47], the first implementation of personalised patient care. It's not simply about making a diagnosis and informing the patient. During the consultation, carers should provide relevant and respectful information to patients, both on the nature of their cancer and on the treatments proposed. This effort is also carried out by an entire care team, no longer just by the patient's general practitioner. Thanks to the formalisation of this process, the situation has changed. Health professionals have now been trained to handle this particular encounter, how to listen and how to convey information that is clear and accessible.

The words have to be spoken, despite the sadness and anguish they will bring. The patient has the right to know. Saying the words eases the tension. Giving a name to the pain, the test results, the chronic fatigue, the unexplained weight loss that has lasted for months. Putting words to this is crucial. You need to be as clear as possible, to speak plainly and simply. This first consultation generates an expectation that is impossible to express. It comes after weeks, sometimes months of latent anxiety, which the patient tries, as best they can, to surmount, to control, to rationalise. The verdict is one the patient is

---

47. "Annonce et accompagnement du diagnostic d'un patient ayant une maladie chronique", *Guide parcours de soin,* Haute Autorité de Santé. Downloadable at the following address <https://www.has-sante.fr/upload/docs/application/pdf/2014 03/guide_annonce_diagnostic_web.pdf>.

anticipating and dreading at the same time, waiting at last to know the nature of the evil that has been gnawing away at them. The wait can't go on. The diagnosis should be made known without too much delay. Establish as calm an atmosphere as possible and say what needs to be said.

Be honest without being brutal – this is the difficult balance you have to find. "You won't have it for much longer". "Get your affairs in order". "Treatments can make you sterile". These kinds of phrases are still uttered to patients today when they have just found out about the disease that has struck them. Although we owe our patients total and straightforward honesty, words can kill. Those kinds of words create an obstacle to the patient's projecting a cure, to the life instinct itself. They can literally kill a patient. Words that explain – even in precise detail – the seriousness of a situation so that it can be understood, these are the words are likely to reassure them.

Avoid being dogmatic

"There's no room for definitive judgement in a medical consultation. I always carefully avoid answering the question 'How long do I have?' Not because I'm afraid to reply, but because I'm a doctor, not a clairvoyant. Of course, there are statistics. Some cancers are treated more successfully than others, and that's a fact. One of my patients, let's call him Henri, defied these statistics. This rather elderly gentleman had cancer that had spread to his whole body. He had a great deal of family support, and despite everything he remained serene in a way that was inspiring. He was especially focused on one thing: that his chemotherapy

sessions not interfere with his bridge games. So we followed a treatment protocol for several months that allowed him to continue playing bridge regularly. After a while, he had to be placed in palliative care because the treatments had not succeeded in stopping the spread of cancer cells in his body.
Always extremely well cared for by his wife and daughters, this man had completed his treatment and was preparing for his death. Then, he recovered, little by little. Against all odds, his cancer went into recession. The cancer process, which in his case had been considered irreversible, was gradually coming to a halt. Every day that passed, his condition improved.
Henri is not alone in this story. Every day, there are patients who defy the odds. Statistics are only statistics. They reflect a general reality. That's why I prefer to focus on life. As long as there is life, there is hope. The sometimes dizzying speed at which medicine is progressing in the field of cancerology should also impose humility on us about our ability to give prognoses."

Alain Toledano

Medical truth is not human truth. We make a diagnosis and give a prognosis based on relevant statistics. But this doesn't necessarily correspond to the way in which people perceive themselves, nor is it an absolute medical truth. Henri's story illustrates this. What counts during the crucial diagnosis announcement is putting aside your certainties as a doctor to see the person facing you. There is often a distortion in communication between on the one hand, technical and scientific language and a medical conception of time, and on the other, an emotional language fraught with fear, patients dealing with their lives and who are at a specific stage of acceptance.

The rhythm of this consultation needs to be in line with the emotions the patient is experiencing. There's no one right way to do this. The only important thing is to be in accord with the person in front of you. Some patients will feel reassured by a doctor who is authoritative and extremely technical; it makes them feel taken care of. The main thing is to be able to choose, and to do it consciously.

When patients feel too anxious, when their desire for projection is too strong, you need to slow the rhythm, slow your speech, but also to make sure the information you are conveying is adapted to your patient. Take the time to explain the care protocol and each stage of the cancer journey in detail, and give the patient time to assimilate this information.

Most often, when a cancer diagnosis is announced, patients are in a state of shock. They are no longer themselves. Psychologically they have changed, and they also have to prepare for physical change. That is a tremendous amount to handle. In opposition to this immobility, we need to set a vital energy in motion. It may seem paradoxical to give momentum to a positive dynamic just as a potentially fatal disease is announced, but this should be done as soon as possible, because the announcement is also the prelude to reconstruction. Not everything is focused on the cancer diagnosis itself. It's essential to talk about recovery at the same time, to define a care plan rather than taking a break before developing the chosen strategy to deal with the cancer. The announcement should also offer the patient some perspective and a way to cope with the disease.

It's often necessary to return to this several times. A state of shock can prevent patients from taking the full measure of what is happening to them and from fully understanding the strategy you are proposing. For this reason, the announcement no longer relies on a single practitioner but on the entire care team that will take care of a patient. Here again, the importance of having multidisciplinary teams working together in a coordinated manner becomes perfectly clear. Everyone knows what the patient has been told, the patient's condition and how the news was received, and based on that knowledge can make a sensitive and useful contribution to helping the patient.

Taking ownership of your own care project

Until the turn of the millennium, patients often followed protocols while remaining unaware of the expected duration of the treatment. Others were prescribed extremely invasive or aggressive treatments or surgery to prevent a risk of recurrence but without further explanation. Medical knowledge has evolved considerably over the last twenty years, but that alone does not explain this kind of negligence on the part of healthcare providers. This abysmal lack of information sharing drove legislators in France to establish the 2002 Patient Rights Act, known as the "Kouchner law", ensuring patients, which insured patients' right to information and to informed consent regarding their treatment.

Despite the significant progress made over the last twenty years, too many patients still follow treatment protocols they have certainly understood are useful but which they know nothing about. But patient information is the first building block in co-creating the care pathway. It's the first element that prevents patients from being totally passive in their treatment, from being objectified and feeling distanced from their own bodies, and it's essential to give them the means to understand their disease and what is being planned to deal with it.

Giving complete information to patients means getting to know them. You have to take their personality, their beliefs and their environment into account, to be able to judge their capacity to listen to what is being conveyed to them. This is closely linked to their emotional state, which should also be taken into account. The empathy that is so essential to the doctor/carer relationship takes on an additional dimension here. This dimension will facilitate a dialogue and a shared information exchange that will benefit everyone, patients and doctors alike.

Giving the patient space

"One of my patients was referred to me by the surgeon who had performed her mastectomy after she was diagnosed with breast cancer. She had the surgery but was adamant about not undergoing any other treatments, especially not chemotherapy.

Her sense of personal freedom was very strong; she could not bear to have anything forced on her, not even a life-saving cancer treatment. In addition, the fear of side effects and the negative effect it would have on her image and appearance seemed unbearable to her. Chemotherapy right away identifies you as a cancer patient, and hair loss makes it apparent. In her mind, it was a symbol that would end up defining her indicating and she refused to accept it.

Still, she agreed for her doctor to schedule an appointment with an oncologist. When she arrived in my office, the diagnosis had already been announced, but I was not aware that she had refused treatment. I explained in detail the steps of her care journey, then asked her how she felt. 'I'm not sure I agree to undergo such a powerful treatment', she answered, then explained that her doctor had been hoping I would convince her to accept. She asked me for a waiting period to think about it.

It's uncommon for doctors to accept such a request; we usually prefer to start treatment as quickly as possible to avoid giving the disease the time to spread.... But while I was taken aback, I proposed she take ten days to think things over. Ten days to make a conscious choice, to become the architect of her own care pathway. She told me later that the trust I showed in giving her this freedom, led to her accepting the treatment because she no longer felt like a passive patient. She felt empowered, and had become the decision maker."

Alain Toledano

The urgency of the situation does not always allow this type of freedom. It's sometimes indispensable to go as quickly as possible, to rush forward, leaving the patients to cope with their distress. But it's always possible later to initiate or resume the dialogue you weren't able to have at first. It's always necessary to understand the anxieties a patient feels.

A specific relationship with the body, a previous death in the family from cancer or other specific situations should be considered. This is the only way to provide the patient with appropriate explanations and answers, and that is what informing the patient is all about. Whether or not a trust relationship is established will have an impact on the patient's experience of the disease. If patients are convinced that the defined treatment plan will be successful, they will accept a treatment and its side effects more easily. They will understand and anticipate them rather than just being afraid. Through maieutics, by explaining the situation clearly and simply, patients can be gradually led to call for their treatment, to become actors in it.

Because the goal here is to give patients the tools they need to understand their disease and to actively participate in their recovery. Patients need to be fully aware of their health status, the disease's progress and the risks it involves. This is the prerequisite for a good understanding of the care protocol. It allows us to define a therapeutic strategy for treating the cancer, objectives that should be determined together. By giving patients all the information involved in their treatment pathway, we give them tools they will use better themselves than if they were used on them by someone else.

In medical jargon, this is called "therapeutic education", the art of giving patients the necessary skills to best manage their own medical treatments and follow them correctly. This term appeared when the number of chronic diseases was increasing and treatments were evolving. Over time, patients needing long-term care no longer had to be hospitalised for every medical intervention but became capable of self-managing their treatments, even aggressive ones. They had to be trained to understand their treatment so that they could take responsibility for them. In 1998, the WHO defined therapeutic education as a means of "helping the patient and his family to acquire knowledge and competencies on the disease and its treatment, in order to better collaborate with the caregivers, and to improve his quality of life".

Beyond the knowledge conveyed by healthcare providers, patients with chronic diseases have experiential knowledge of their disease. This knowledge is valuable and should be seen as legitimate expertise in the context of the care relationship. This, too, enables a partnership to be established between doctor and patient. If we are attentive to the patient's personal knowledge of their own body and their experience of the disease – expertise that the doctor does not possess – we can co-create the level of prescription, adapting the patient's course of treatment according to their difficulties and needs.

Taking the time to listen to patients and hear about their side effects allows us to adapt the treatment accordingly: extend it, reduce it, prescribe drugs to help improve digestion, relieve headaches, ease pain.... We can always adapt. Treatments are not necessarily set in stone. The dose of a chemotherapy drug can be reduced, and treatment can be made outside a doctor's office or hospital, on vacation for example, to give patients a kind of respiration.

If a treatment is too unbearable, patients might not follow it, or might follow it poorly. Giving patients control over their treatment not only makes it bearable but effective. In general, there is no compliance (the act of following and respecting a medical prescription) when there is no adherence to the care plan. And if you don't understand the issues, you can't adhere to the plan.

Nutrition and hormone therapy

"Having a nutritionist is clearly useful in managing the changes in weight patients experience when they have cancer, and it can help them adopt new eating habits that they will maintain long afterwards. But we also see additional benefits. Many types of breast cancer require hormonal treatment several years after chemo and radiation. It's not a very aggressive treatment, just oral tablets, but the medication makes you gain weight. Over time, many women are bothered by the weight gain and stop taking their pills. The nutritionists can help patients before this happens by discussing their eating habits, talking about the reasons for the weight gain and explaining the effects of hormones, giving them the tools to minimize the weight gain without stopping them from living their lives. This means our patients are more conscientious about respecting their hormone therapy treatments. This significantly limits the risk of recurrence, and they learn to accept it without suffering negative consequences."

Alain Toledano

People often use the term empowerment to describe the new role being given to patients – they now have greater control over the decisions made affecting their health. The doctor is no longer the only one in charge. This is the very vocation of integrative medicine, to make the patient a full-fledged actor in the care process and increase patient participation. If we are doing everything possible to offer patients the tools they can use to improve their quality of life, to feel better, they should also be directly involved in their treatment and their recovery. In this situation, it's also easier for them to articulate the difficulties they are experiencing since they know solutions can be proposed.

Beyond the treatment protocol in the strictest sense, a patient's behaviour has a major influence on healing. Alcohol, smoking, nutrition, physical activity – all these factors have a profound impact on a patient's recovery. Co-creating the care pathway is crucial. It's unthinkable to confine yourself to a moralising and prescriptive stance. On the contrary, patients should be given the keys to understanding the impact of those behaviours and the means to act on them. This is the only way to engage patients in a process of sustainable change, and the meaning itself of integrative medicine.

Conclusion

Making connections that elevate us

"Each patient has something to offer us. As doctors, our exchanges constantly nourish our thinking and our practice, and my encounter with Min was no exception. Her cancer journey was very much in keeping with how I believe we should treat patients. Her determination to engage fully in her care programme and to understand the issues and objectives was influential not only for her but also for us as her carers.

The most important thing I have retained is the life force that music gave her during that time. Music enabled her to hold onto her vital energy throughout her cancer journey, to find the thread that connected her to life and grab onto it.

It was very meaningful for us to share her experience with as many people as possible, because music is also generous. Thanks to the altruism inherent in music, perhaps others can also live better with cancer."

Alain Toledano

Because that is what this book is all about: hope and life. Through what music can teach us and through our own personal experience as patient, musician and doctor, we wanted to show that it's possible to keep on living during and after cancer, that it's possible to protect yourself despite the aggressiveness and invasiveness of the disease and its treatment. Once humanity has been restored, the disease stops monopolising your life, stops taking up all the space.

Music is deeply human; it's part of what defines us as people. That's why it plays such a special role in our lives. It offers tangible support. Min's experience shows us that it's possible to continue living and enjoying life after cancer. The power of music helped her and carried her through the ordeal, just as it transported millions of people during the recent health crisis. You don't have to be a professional musician to experience the benefits of music; it's there for all of us. Music can be a vital anchor in the face of adversity.

Music is obviously not the only option for living well with cancer; it can be as simple as keeping up a regular bridge game during treatment. In the end, it doesn't matter what you grab onto – what matters is to keep living. We've tried to show that this is possible despite the disease, its side effects and the difficulties it engenders. From complementary care to the way we engage in the care relationship, every step counts. Every step helps keep hope alive while you're struggling with disease.

There's always room for hope. Medical progress is evolving in extraordinary ways, and more and more types of cancer are being treated with increasing success. Social progress is leading to more patient-centred care, which is only fitting. There's still progress to be made, and the goal of this book is also to give patients and their families the tools to assert their rights and take ownership of their care. Cancer is an ordeal that forever transforms the people who've gone through it. You don't come out of it quite the same person; you learn about yourself, and life takes on a new meaning. But there's yet another step. There's the re-building, and that's what we have to focus on.

We wanted to close this book with a song that symbolises a feeling of hope and optimism, a powerful life force, and *Over the Rainbow* does just that.

Harold Arlen, *Over the Rainbow*: hope

"This song by Harold Arlen, composed in just one single night, is taken from the film *"The Wizard of Oz"*. It was one of the first full films I saw as a child. I must have been about eight and it remained, for many years, etched in my memory. This little girl, transported into this motley and multi-coloured universe, really made an impact on me as a child.

The unconditional friendship that is forged between Dorothy, the heroine, and the three slightly flawed characters, the cowardly lion, the tin man and the scarecrow, is a wonderful fable that illustrates the importance of friendship. It had a very special meaning for me during my cancer.

I see this song as a pure embodiment of hope. By its key, in E flat major, but also through the lyrics, and of course the memories that lie within me. For as long as I can remember, I've always come back to this song for hope and inspiration. It tells us we can find a place where 'skies are blue' and 'leave the clouds far behind'. It tells us it's possible to reach that joyful, colourful world. Maybe this seems childish, but it's precisely that childish simplicity that makes me feel optimistic, that reassures me, the idea that we can have joy in life for tomorrow. It ultimately gives us a reason to live.

Min-Jung Kym

Table

Achevé d'imprimer en septembre 2023
par la Sté ACORT Europe
www.cogetefi.com

Dépôt légal à parution

Imprimé en France